New Orleans Women and the Poydras Home

NEW ORLEANS
WOMEN

·····— AND THE —·····

POYDRAS HOME

MORE DURABLE THAN MARBLE

PAMELA TYLER

LOUISIANA STATE UNIVERSITY PRESS

BATON ROUGE

To Anne Firor Scott,
my favorite pioneer

Published by Louisiana State University Press
Copyright © 2016 by Louisiana State University Press
All rights reserved
Manufactured in the United States of America
First printing

Designer: Michelle A. Neustrom
Typeface: Sina Nova
Printer and binder: Maple Press

LIBRARY OF CONGRESS CATALOGING-IN-PUBLICATION DATA

Names: Tyler, Pamela.
Title: New Orleans women and the Poydras Home : more durable than marble /
   Pamela Tyler.
Description: Baton Rouge : Louisiana State University Press, 2016. | Includes
   bibliographical references and index.
Identifiers: LCCN 2015042800| ISBN 978-0-8071-6322-1 (cloth : alkaline paper) |
   ISBN 978-0-8071-6323-8 (pdf) | ISBN 978-0-8071-6324-5 (epub) | ISBN 978-0-807-1-6325-2
   (mobi)
Subjects: LCSH: Poydras Home (New Orleans, La.) —History. |
   Charities—Louisiana—New Orleans—History. | Women
   philanthropists—Louisiana—New Orleans—History. |
   Orphanages—Louisiana—New Orleans—History. | Poor girls—Services
   for—Louisiana—New Orleans—History. | Retirement
   communities—Louisiana—New Orleans—History. | Congregate
   housing—Louisiana—New Orleans—History. | New Orleans (La.) —Social
   conditions.
Classification: LCC HV99.N42 P687 2016 | DDC 362.73/2—dc23 LC record available at
   http://lccn.loc.gov/2015042800

CONTENTS

Illustrations follow page 86.

PREFACE

hance arguably plays a larger role than choice in the course of human events; history is littered with indirect linkages. A prime example is the chain of events that led to the establishment of a home for orphaned and indigent girls in the turbulent city of New Orleans in 1817. This institution, the Poydras Asylum, which endured for nearly a century and a half as a refuge for girls who needed a home and which eventually served several thousand young people, owes its start to some seemingly random and unconnected events. Over the decades, this institution survived bank failures, the Union army's occupation, the turmoil of Reconstruction, bitter religious dissension, a crippling economic depression, two world wars, a catastrophic hurricane, and deadly epidemics of yellow fever, cholera, and influenza. In the mid-twentieth century, as the rise of foster care began to render orphans' institutionalization obsolete, the individuals who operated the asylum made a decision to alter their mission, and in 1959 the Poydras Home was reborn to serve the elderly.

This volume tells two stories. One is the story of an institution that has served so many, so well, for so long. The other is the tale of a small coterie of New Orleans women, the unpaid board of managers of Poydras. It was they who created the institution, nurtured it, financed it, managed it, and, on more than one occasion, saved it. In some years, they fought merely to maintain their operation; in others, they expanded to pursue new goals. They were no strangers to ridicule and skepticism, particularly in the early years when they challenged ideas about gender propriety. The cast of characters changed over the years as Death claimed his due, but new managers were found. Learning competence and courage from veterans, they ensured continuity and carried the ideals and vision of the founders forward across the decades. The Poydras

Home continues to operate as it began two hundred years ago, under the direction of a volunteer board of managers, who, to this day, are all women.

What follows is an institutional history in narrative form. From voluminous records, I have constructed a chronological story and added analysis and perspective. My colleagues in the history profession will note that this book is not particularly "thesis-driven." But that observation really underscores the fact that the central theme is glaringly familiar, repeated in various histories again and again: the story of unpaid women, accustomed to the concept of benevolence and motivated by their religion, undertaking a mission of charity, facing innumerable challenges, exercising executive skills, encountering formidable setbacks, but ultimately succeeding. Like most white women involved in voluntary associations, the women of Poydras were, for most of their two-century history, traditionalists in terms of class and race. In their own words, in document after document, they left behind a record that details both their unconscious elitism and their genuine compassion, intelligence, and accomplishments. Always striving to do good for others, Poydras managers of past decades were a combination of often contradictory qualities. Imperfect though they were, they set themselves to an admirable task, and they prevailed.

The Poydras Home of today has an annual operating budget of $7.5 million and a staff numbering 140. Its board manages a multi-million-dollar portfolio of assets. When the home began in Phoebe Hunter's drawing room on a cold January day in 1817, not only was its success uncertain, but the women who sipped tea and hatched plans had no money, only an idea. This volume will trace the genesis and flowering of that idea.

ACKNOWLEDGMENTS

The convoluted process of birthing this book involved a long gestation period. Between the embryonic idea and a fully formed manuscript lies a great deal of help, and I take keen pleasure in acknowledging here and now those who aided me.

After Hurricane Katrina and the subsequent ordeal New Orleans endured, I interviewed many women whose efforts were advancing the sluggish recovery of a great city. I later published articles about their work and occasionally spoke to audiences about the female face of recovery in the Crescent City. In 2008, Ruthie Frierson, whose Citizens for 1 Greater New Orleans performed herculean work to forever change the status quo for the better, invited me to address a gathering of local activist women, speaking broadly on the history of women's work for reform in New Orleans.

As I enjoyed post-lecture conversation in the comfortable space of the New Orleans Lawn Tennis Club, a stranger approached. She guided me toward a broad expanse of windows and pointed across the courts toward a complex of roseate stucco buildings, the Poydras Home. That was my first encounter with Pat Rosamond, a past president of the Poydras Home's board of managers and the dynamic chair of a committee established to find an author for a proposed bicentennial history of their redoubtable institution. In the course of our brief talk, a seed was planted. The book committee—Catherine Edwards, Pat Rosamond, Nelda Sibley, Karen Smith, and the late Betsy Ewing—ultimately decided that I would be the proper scholar to tackle the long history of their cherished facility. I thank them for their wisdom in knowing that a history should be written, for their willingness to give me *carte blanche* access to the voluminous Poydras records (usually kept under restriction in

Special Collections at Tulane University), and, most of all, for their confidence in me through a long journey.

Former Poydras board member Mary Langlois shared a massive cache of documents regarding the ambitious expansion of Poydras in the 1990s, which were terrifically helpful. To the many other board members, the Poydras staff members, and the former residents of Poydras who sat for interviews with me, a big thank you; I could not have written this history without your input.

Sally Kenney, director of the Newcomb College Institute, made it possible for me to have a full year in New Orleans with only light academic duties. By naming me the Dora Bonquois Ellis Visiting Historian in 2012, the NCI made me a researcher-in-residence, thus allowing me twelve months away from my position at the University of Southern Mississippi, a year I spent plowing through reams of handwritten ledgers, volumes of minutes, and stacks of correspondence from years gone by. What a luxury. I owe a debt of gratitude to Sally and to all the staff at the Newcomb College Institute, and in particular to Bea Calvert, librarian at Newcomb's Vorhoff Library; Susan Tucker, the Vorhoff's longtime archivist; and Jaelle Scheuerman, information technology specialist.

Since I routinely spent six to seven hours a day, five days each week, in the hushed reading room of Tulane's Special Collections, I often joked that the staff should simply cut a key for me and allow me to come and go at will. That they would not do, but on all of my other requests for help they delivered. Every researcher knows her debt to skilled librarians and archivists, and I am no different. Leon Miller, head, was from the start interested in my project, encouraging and accommodating in every way. His staff fetched boxes and volumes and frequently pointed me to other relevant sources. In particular, I appreciate Sean Benjamin's high level of competence. He must hold the record for mastery of New Orleans history by a Canadian transplant. While researching at the Archives of the Archdiocese of New Orleans, I found in Dorenda Dupont an extraordinary level of helpfulness; she guided me to pertinent documents with pleasant efficiency and, after ascertaining my focus, suggested other sources that proved to be just what I needed.

I am most fortunate in belonging to a collective of women historians, from four states in the region, who meet twice yearly to read and critique each other's work, always with rigor and the leavening of good humor. Accordingly, I thank the Delta Women Writers (you know who you are) for their feedback on a portion of this work; their suggestions and comments were, as ever, perceptive and valuable.

To all the scholars who have researched and written about aspects of New Orleans, your rich scholarship has guided me. Particularly as I groped my way toward understanding developments of the nineteenth century in this city, I relied on your works. I take such pleasure in being among your number.

Clarence Mohr deserves special praise for kindly interrupting his own important work to read and critique this manuscript, which he did with his usual thoroughness and insight. I appreciate his input very much.

Alisa Plant, now editor-in-chief at the University of Nebraska Press, believed in this project from the start and did much to encourage me that I could appeal to two audiences, both scholars and the general public. Her enthusiasm and confidence meant a great deal. Her colleague at the Press, Catherine Kadair, proved to be a discerning copy editor who deployed her skills to very good effect.

No doubt, deficiencies and omissions remain, but they are in no way a reflection upon those who helped me so generously when I asked.

My partner Leslie Parr, a notable historian who by now has heard a very great deal about the Poydras Home, sustains me by her willingness to hear still more. She gamely read every word of this manuscript with her sharp editorial pencil in hand, much to my benefit. Even better, she delights me by her eagerness to learn, consume, and experience all things New Orleans with me.

As I close this project, I look back across the years, to the Poydras managers from another era. Clad in voluminous dresses that covered them from neck to wrists to the tops of their morocco leather shoes, barred by law and custom from opportunities and pathways that twenty-first-century women take for granted, those early managers showed dedication, uncommon good sense, and vision. In the pages that follow, I will tell you what they did and how they did it. This telling is possible only because of their foresight in painstakingly preserving records for posterity. Their papers are an absolute treasure trove for the historian—exactly, I think, as the women of the Poydras board anticipated they would be some day.

For a final thought, I turn to Dorothy Parker. When asked about her enjoyment of writing, the divine Dottie told her interviewer tartly, "I do not like writing. I like *having written*." Amen, Miss Parker, amen.

New Orleans Women and the Poydras Home

ORPHANS AND ORPHANAGES
A Historical Overview

Old Mother Hubbard went to the cupboard
To give her poor doggy a bone;
But when she got there, the cupboard was bare,
And so the poor doggy had none.

Poor little Oliver Twist, so thin and slight, appealing with his empty bowl for "more." Poor little Jane Eyre, alone and friendless. Young Heidi, cast away among strangers, yearning for her mountains. Pollyanna, Harry Potter—orphans all. Classic novels present us with memorable portraits of woebegone children, bereft of their parents by dreadful strokes of misfortune and forced to endure pangs of suffering while in the custody of uncaring adults. The most distressing circumstances emerge on the pages wherein the youngsters are sent into institutional care. In orphanages and workhouses, the reader encounters the bleakest of scenarios—cheerless buildings, fireless grates, thin gruel, and pathologically cruel staff who, regularly and with alacrity, cuff, whip, mock, deprive, and shame their pathetic little charges.

Cultural stereotypes from literature have a powerful grip on our collective imaginations. Before beginning this account of the Poydras Asylum, as this refuge for homeless and needy girls was known for most of its years, a respect for truth demands going beyond the pages of Charles Dickens and Charlotte Brontë and into the historian's realm for a basic understanding of orphans and orphanages. What follows in this brief chapter is fact from a historian, not fiction from a novelist.

A popular and traditional view of the nineteenth-century United States tends to emphasize several stirring themes of success: the war to preserve the

Union and emancipate four million enslaved people; the pioneers' triumphant westward expansion; the rise of big business, yielding great fortunes and a steadily improving standard of living. Too often overlooked in a superficial summary of the century is one of its darkest sides, the grinding poverty that stalked victims in every city, town, and hamlet. The life of a laborer, whether in mill, mine, shop, or field, was precarious; steady, year-round employment eluded all but the most fortunate. Seasonal work stoppages meant chronic unemployment or underemployment for many, while waves of arriving immigrants created fierce competition for even the most brutally demanding jobs. With no regulatory legislation to govern the workplace, employers freely subjected workers to long hours, low pay, and dangerous conditions. Unions, tragically weak in the face of employer and government hostility, served perhaps 4 percent of the working class as the nineteenth century ended, meaning that most workers had little leverage to protect themselves from exploitation. Six-day workweeks were the norm, and the concept of a "weekend" lay far in the future. Exhausted workers, routinely handling dangerous machinery and toxic chemicals, were at all times vulnerable to pay cuts and layoffs. "The iron law of wages" meant that employers felt justified in paying as little as possible, and if a man or woman rebelled against the meager pay offered, a surplus of labor ensured that there would always be another to take his or her place.

Among the laboring classes, very few men reliably earned a "family wage," that is, a steady income sufficient to support wife and children fully. Consequently, supplementary cash income generated by wives and children completed the financial foundation of working-class families. Many a wife took in washing or sewed for the public; many women labored to shelter, cook, and wash for complete strangers in return for a small weekly sum from those boarders. Poor women did piecework at home and peddled on the streets; they scavenged for coal by the railroad tracks, foraged for berries and plums along fencerows, and counted pennies spent in the market. Children sold newspapers and flowers, shined shoes, ran errands. A family's livelihood ebbed and flowed with circumstances: a new baby temporarily took away a wife's ability to earn; a child entering adolescence could be withdrawn from school and put to work; one adult male might earn a pay raise while another took a pay cut. It was a sink-or-swim world, stunning for its sheer lack of safeguards: no workmen's compensation, no wage-and-hour laws, no unemployment insurance, no laws to protect health and safety. Such a world created terrific uncertainty for all; everyone was vulnerable to misfortune. Although belief in upward mobility was strong in this land of opportunity, and some workers did manage to put by a little money or buy a modest home, the lives of the poor were shockingly hard and always precarious; nothing more than luck stood between many of them and economic disaster.

How much more vulnerable, then, were those families diminished by the death of a parent. Throughout the entire nineteenth century, average life expectancy in the United States never topped forty-eight years for men or women. Early death lurked in myriad circumstances. Working men in their prime succumbed in industrial accidents in coal mines, foundries, and lumber mills, in railroad disasters and steamboat explosions. They expired from infectious diseases; they died from sheer overwork and poor nutrition. Women, consigned to lives of backbreaking domestic work without benefit of labor-saving devices and facing repeated childbirths in an era of unregulated fertility, often proved unable to withstand the consequences of inadequate nutrition and hard work coupled with poor obstetrical care. As a chilling consequence, the average woman faced a one-in-thirty chance of being a maternal mortality statistic in the nineteenth century.

With no margin for misfortune, every poor family that lost a parent suffered immediately. Poor women left with children were especially pathetic in their widowhood. Not all women left alone with children were widows, of course; some were deserted, some were divorced, some had never married. But all single mothers, beyond a fortunate few, needed to earn. Options for women's work were circumscribed by ideas about gender, and most jobs were frankly closed to women. When they could find employment, women who suddenly needed to earn faced a grim reality of drawing one-third to one-half of men's wages. Society generally supported this harsh situation; a widely accepted notion held that women did not belong in the workforce and should instead be supported by a male breadwinner while they devoted themselves to marriage, motherhood, and domesticity.

As the nation began its inexorable shift from rural to urban, ties to family and community were often stretched and broken. In an increasingly transient age, many of the poor in cities lacked bonds to kin, friends, church, or community. Consider the case of a single mother, whether widowed, deserted, divorced, or never married, newly arrived in an urban setting. If deprived of an extended family or trusted neighbors, a working-class woman in the city, left alone with her young children, might have no one to turn to for help with childcare. If work became available to her, she faced a cruel choice: neglect her children in order to earn as a scrub woman or factory hand, or forgo wages to stay home and care for her young family. Succeeding at earning meant failing at parenting, a distressing paradox. (Of course, if death claimed a *mother,* the surviving spouse would likely have a job but little ability to deal with domestic responsibilities, yet a man who buried his wife could count on sympathetic understanding about his inability to manage a household. Ideas about gender being what they were, no one expected a man to work all day and then face cooking a meal, cleaning a house, and caring for children in the evenings.)

Difficult circumstances well short of the death of a spouse could also plunge a household into chaos. Bouts of illness frequently rendered adults weak and sick, facing slow and uncertain convalescence. Addiction to alcohol, opium, or gambling could leave an adult, male or female, unable to contribute to the household's welfare. Desertion, essentially a poor man's divorce, was certainly not an uncommon phenomenon, nor was unwed motherhood. Some people were improvident; others unlucky. For a multiplicity of reasons, many a nineteenth-century household could not reliably meet the needs of all its members.

Early America inherited its ideas about alms for the poor from England, where "poor laws" provided assistance to paupers in the form of "outdoor relief." Local governments doled out skimpy stipends to the "deserving" poor in times of greatest need, in order to allow poverty-stricken individuals to continue living "outdoors," that is, in the community, in their own quarters. In return for scant stipends, the poor, if physically able, were expected to work, the men often chopping in municipal wood yards, the women stitching in community sewing rooms. On the other hand, the "undeserving" poor could expect to receive nothing; righteous communities judged that the wages of drunkenness, sexual immorality, or laziness should be poverty. Over time, local governments in the United States evolved systems offering help for paupers in the form of "indoor relief." This meant care in an institution known as the "poorhouse," a word that evoked disgrace. Early on, the county poorhouse, almost always operating on a mere shoestring of a budget, promiscuously housed not only the desperately poor of the community but also orphaned children and the mentally ill. However, an enlightened nineteenth-century citizenry (and enlightenment is certainly a relative term in this context) gradually built separate facilities to house orphans and the insane.

Eventually, the orphanage emerged as the most popular answer to the problem of childcare for distressed and struggling adults of either sex (although usually women). Certainly, orphan asylums housed destitute children who had lost both parents and who had no relatives willing or able to take them in, but the crucial fact to understand in considering orphanages is that, as the nineteenth century progressed, more and more children in them had one and sometimes both parents living. The so-called "half orphan" was a familiar presence in institutional care, as was the child with two living but impoverished parents who could no longer provide a home. While going to the poorhouse inflicted a stigma, approaching an orphanage did not, and so the poor consciously used orphanages to meet their needs in rough times. Many an adult deposited children into the asylum with the firm intent of reclaiming them when a crisis had passed. The records of any nineteenth-century orphanage will reveal a constant churning of admissions and withdrawals; the average length of stay for many children was under one year. "Orphanages" were asylums in the most literal sense—refuges from harsh circumstances, safe shelters from the exigencies that often buffeted Americans and destabilized families in that era before social welfare services.

Although local governments funded poorhouses, orphanages of the nineteenth century were almost always private and sectarian. Religion motivated many individuals to establish homes for children in need; in American cities, Protestant, Catholic, and Jewish congregations founded children's homes as symbols of religious pride. All strove to shelter, feed, clothe, and educate the children placed in their care, while also giving moral instruction consistent with their particular religious faith. Middle-class Protestant women established numerous asylums in the antebellum years, and beginning in the 1830s, the rapid growth of the nation's Catholic population spurred the creation of Catholic asylums.

The quality of services provided varied widely. Dependent as they were on subscriptions, donations, and legacies, sectarian children's institutions saw their revenue shrink with every economic downturn that pinched the general populace. Most asylums tried to collect some payment toward a half-orphan's upkeep from the surviving parent and did not hesitate to press fathers and mothers who turned up on visiting days. They also sought and frequently obtained appropriations from city and state governments to help them with their mission.

We will never know the percentage of Americans who spent a portion of their childhood in orphanages, but it is safe to say that, in the nineteenth century, it was considerable. Historian Timothy Hacsi notes that there were far more orphan asylums than reformatories and that, from the Civil War through the Depression, more dependent children were cared for in orphanages than by any other means. After an interlude of life among strangers at the asylum, most children returned to their birth families if conditions improved at home. Some, however, remained in institutional care until they "aged out" and were released to begin life on the outside, usually around age sixteen. Still others were "placed out," or apprenticed, to learn skills that would allow them to become self-supporting in adulthood. Age at "binding out" varied greatly, and boys outnumbered girls in this practice.

The family taking in a child from the asylum as an apprentice agreed to shelter, feed, and clothe the orphan, plus teach a skill; in return, the child labored in the family. No doubt there were unscrupulous, unfeeling individuals who took children only for the labor they could get, but families generally offered children the lessons necessary for becoming responsible, self-supporting adults, in the setting of a genuine home. Though recognizing that some children might be exploited, asylum managers, by placing children in families, hoped to build skill sets and character traits that would ensure self-sufficiency in adulthood. Furthermore, the discharge of older children via placement in families opened orphanage spaces and allowed admission of younger, more defenseless and vulnerable children into the asylum, a calculation that must have guided many decisions at overcrowded institutions.

After the Civil War, the practice of "placing out" declined steeply. According to progressive reformer Homer Folks, an early social worker and well-known student of orphanages, by 1875 the indenture system had "passed largely into disuse, if not into disrepute."[1] By late century, more struggling parents than ever were using asylums as a temporary measure, with most making modest, if irregular, payments for their children's upkeep. Children admitted in these circumstances were not eligible for placing out so long as someone made an effort to contribute financially, even if only intermittently. It is not stretching a point to observe that the orphanage functioned in many cases as a virtual boarding school for the poor.

Orphanages became steadily more humane as time passed. Children in institutional care were clearly not to blame for their needy condition. Other institutions for the poor, such as the poorhouse and the prison, deliberately meted out harsh treatment to inmates, but children's asylums, where a majority of inmates had families to whom they hoped to return, existed to protect and nurture innocent children. By the twentieth century, realizing that they were ill equipped to help children with special needs, asylums increasingly weeded out youngsters with severe problems, such as blindness, epilepsy, paralysis, or developmental delays. Sending children such as these to specialized facilities, which were becoming available in cities, accomplished the goal of allowing an orphanage to care for a population of needy or neglected children possessed of normal physical and mental abilities and thus to create a fairly normal "home," albeit a home with upwards of one hundred children in its family.

The dawn of the twentieth century witnessed a significant shift in philosophies about orphanages. The *Delineator,* a widely circulated magazine for middle-class women, launched a zealous "child rescue" campaign under the editorial leadership of celebrated author Theodore Dreiser. Printing poignant stories of needy or neglected children in every issue for almost four years, the popular magazine urged foster care for the inmates of orphanages and warned that a lonely, unloved child would become a troubled, and perhaps troublesome, adult; warm testimonials from adoptive mothers gave added weight. After Dreiser cannily interested Theodore Roosevelt in his crusade, the president convened a pivotal meeting, the White House Conference on Dependent Children.[2] Meeting in January 1909, the gathering attracted some well-known child advocates, among them Jane Addams, Jacob Riis, Lillian Wald, Homer Folks, Booker T. Washington, and Dreiser himself, as well as enthusiastic child welfare supporters and earnest representatives of charitable organizations, some two hundred in all. Those assembled heard lectures, attended panel discussions, and exchanged information. Ultimately they reached an important consensus, overwhelmingly agreeing that children should never be placed in an orphanage merely because a family was poverty-stricken. They voiced the particular criticism that orphanages stifled individualism with regimentation and produced "institutional" children unfit for adulthood.

Convinced that life in a large, anonymous group had pernicious effects on children, these elite progressive reformers rallied behind three alternatives. Most preferable in their eyes was payment of "mothers' pensions," stipends allowing financially distressed but "respectable" women to keep their children with them despite hard times. A second acceptable option involved finding foster homes in the community for children who needed them, and a third solution, put forward in case mothers' pensions and foster care did not materialize, posited making institutional life for children more palatable. This last alternative involved organizing an asylum into the "cottage system," housing small groups of perhaps ten to twenty children in separate buildings with housemothers, to allow for more "homelike" conditions.

Above all, the 1909 White House conferees soundly repudiated large congregate orphanages as solutions for the care of neglected or destitute children. The group's report to Theodore Roosevelt stated emphatically:

> Home life is the highest and finest product of civilization. Children should not be deprived of it except for urgent and compelling reasons. Children of parents of worthy character, suffering from temporary misfortune and children of reasonably efficient and deserving mothers who are without the support of the normal breadwinner, should, as a rule, be kept with their parents, such aid being given as may be necessary to maintain suitable homes for the rearing of the children . . . preferably in the form of private charity, rather than of public relief. Except in unusual circumstances, the home should not be broken up for reasons of poverty, but only for considerations of inefficiency or immorality.[3]

Of course, ideas floated by well-intentioned child welfare workers in the rarified setting of the White House did not immediately affect actual practices in local communities, and new congregate orphanages did in fact continue to be built for quite some time after 1909. However, this watershed meeting signaled that change was on the way. The rise of psychology as a discipline began to yield studies and findings about child development that supported the policies progressives had advocated at the conference. Impressed with theories of personality development, some orphanages slowly began to offer children more opportunities for activities "off campus," in the community and with other children beyond the institution. The result was more outings—to circuses, minstrel shows, and moving pictures—and more interactions with other children, in Scout troops, summer camps, and athletic leagues. By this time, most orphanages had already abandoned their own educational systems and were enrolling their children in public schools, although Catholic orphanages notably resisted this trend for quite some time. Ideas emanating from the 1909 White House conference on dependent children gradually filtered into the mainstream and began to act as a centrifugal force, steadily pulling asylum children outward and into the broader community, away from the sheltering and simultaneously confining influence of the orphanage.

The rise of social work as a profession led institutions to depend more and more on outside experts, a situation with significant consequences. If a local institution joined the Community Chest, through which charitable donations were distributed to worthy charities in a community, its facilities underwent a rigorous critique before funds were allocated. Its managers received instructions about upgrading physical plant and personnel, about modifying policies and adjusting routines. Even the rare asylum that did not need Community Chest funds and thus chose not to affiliate with it felt encroachment from other quarters. By the late nineteenth century, states were creating boards of charities and institutions, designed to inspect prisons and asylums and submit annual reports. Though almost all orphanages were private and sectarian, they commonly received city and state stipends to help care for growing numbers of children ordered admitted by juvenile courts; those stipends were increasingly contingent upon satisfactory inspection reports. State inspectors counted beds, noted fire escapes, inquired about dental care, and lifted lids of pots on the stoves to examine the day's dinner in preparation. They demanded that asylum staff submit many kinds of data. Not surprisingly, they encountered resistance from private institutions, but the state's power of the purse usually proved persuasive.

In the nineteenth century, regulations had been almost unheard of, meaning that institutions were, in our present-day view, outrageously free and accountable to no outsiders, but by the twentieth century, that had changed forever. Moreover, orphanages began to hire professional social workers and recreation staff; they kept professional case histories of the children. Gradually they became dependent on outside experts for training their staff, regulating admissions, and setting policies. While this presumably meant progress and benefited the children, it nonetheless caused volunteer boards of managers to trust their own instincts less as they leaned on "experts" more. By mid-twentieth century, a trend had materialized; hiring social workers, activities directors, nursing directors, bookkeepers, psychologists, dieticians, and other professional staff ensured that boards of volunteer managers were increasingly removed from the day-to-day operations of their institutions. They had ceased to "manage" in any literal sense at all, moving instead toward a more familiar business model of setting broad policy but distancing themselves from the routine operations of the institution.

Meanwhile, the progressives' idea that poverty alone should never send children to orphanages motivated a growing cross section of reform-minded citizens to demand mothers' pensions, or stipends for "deserving" impoverished women with children. Although a few outspoken feminist activists argued that mothering was socially useful labor that by its nature entitled women to compensation, the majority of advocates, such as the influential National Congress of Mothers (forerunner of the better-known Parents and Teachers Association, or PTA), took the conservative and utilitarian view that payments to "deserving" mothers who were widowed or deserted would serve society by combatting the twin evils of juvenile delinquency and child labor. Child advocates from well-known settlement houses in Chicago, New York, and Boston endorsed the concept, which was also sold as a cost-saving measure. Referring to a recently widowed woman with five young children, whose eldest was only nine years old, Children's Aid Society literature in Louisiana bluntly posed this practical question: *"Would you rather pay $1,000 a year for institutional care for these children, or $412.80 to keep them with their mother?"* In 1911, the state of Illinois led the way by passing the nation's first bill to award a stipend to impoverished mothers with dependent children. Within the next six years, thirty-four more states adopted similar legislation. The trend continued until, by the time of Franklin Roosevelt's New Deal, only Georgia and South Carolina had failed to embrace some version of the measure.

Mothers' aid was never intended to allow mothers to stay home with their children full-time and enjoy a middle-class lifestyle; authorities who awarded mothers' pensions expected recipients to work, although at "part-time, seasonal, or home work." Mothers' pensions thus never financed a genuinely comfortable standard of living in those early years, but they were usually sufficient to permit a struggling but motivated mother to keep her home afloat and her family intact, if she scrimped, and if she supplemented the niggardly pension with small earnings.[4]

Increasingly, child welfare agencies encouraged poor mothers to follow this course. A resolution passed at the 1930 White House Conference on Children stated the strong preference of children's advocates for protecting and preserving family life rather than offering substitutes for it. These facts meant that the type of child who entered an orphanage changed as the twentieth century unfolded. Because medical advances and rising standards of living had boosted life expectancies, the "full orphan," a child who had neither mother nor father living, was more and more an anomaly. Meanwhile, an impoverished single parent of good character, whether widowed, divorced, or deserted, could look to state aid if she had children to support. In the years after 1911, one after another, the various states began to subsidize the care of impoverished children in their own homes. Seldom did sheer poverty drive needy half orphans into institutional care any longer.

And so another change manifested itself in the orphanage. Instead of full or half orphans, youngsters admitted were often those removed from dysfunctional homes, or "broken homes" as they came to be called. (Authorities set the definitions of "inadequate home" and "unfit mother," and their standards had a definite class bias.) In the nineteenth century, it had been grieving and distressed widows, concerned neighbors, or kindly clergymen who brought orphaned and needy children to the gates of orphanages. But with the proliferation of juvenile courts and public welfare departments in the twentieth century, many children, judged neglected, endangered, or delinquent because of circumstances created by violent, alcoholic, mentally unstable, or otherwise troubled or neglectful parents, entered asylums via the intervention of these intermediary agencies.

Financially enabled by mothers' pensions, sober, law-abiding, but impoverished women who lacked a breadwinner in the household could keep their children at home, but moralistic city and county investigating committees tended to withhold mothers' pensions from women they deemed unworthy.

Originally, when "bad" women (basically women with records of promiscuity, drunkenness, narcotics use, or crime, or women who accepted their poverty too casually, without struggle) faced economic hard times, committees rated them ineligible for the financial aid that would have helped them maintain a home and keep their children. However, by the 1920s, few orphanages refused, as they had refused in the nineteenth century, to accept children of such "unworthy" parents. So, while mothers' aid allowed "good" women to keep their children at home, orphanages increasingly became the place for children of "bad" women, or "unfit mothers," whom local authorities denied pensions.

Still another change in *modus operandi* was apparent. By the early twentieth century, society deemed foster care preferable to care in a congregate institution. Rather than going to the orphanage, the stream of neglected children removed from "unfit mothers" began to flow to foster families who were paid by the state to care for children *en famille*. Because progressive elites had long argued that, far from saving children, large impersonal asylums were creating a cadre of social misfits, they viewed the triumph of the foster care system as a victory for neglected or endangered children.

But emotionally disturbed or traumatized children and poorly socialized children often could not find a place in the foster care system, and so twentieth-century orphanages still performed a function for society. More and more, the so-called "orphanages" sheltered troubled youth with behavioral or psychological problems. The "orphans' home" of the nineteenth century became instead the "group home" of the mid-twentieth, where trained professionals dispensed therapy. As Kenneth Cmiel has shown in his meticulously researched history of a well-known children's institution in Chicago, abnormal psychology gradually began to replace poverty as the key circumstance governing admission to a children's home in the twentieth century.[5] In short, thanks to a confluence of circumstances, the orphanage of old simply became obsolete.

Thus it may be seen that the orphanage, as an institution, was far from static; it underwent profound changes during the nineteenth and twentieth centuries as ideas about children's needs shifted. Dynamic situations called for flexibility and wise reactions on the part of those who managed children's homes; adapting to change was essential for institutional survival. The trends described in this chapter buffeted the Female Orphan Asylum of New Orleans and presented challenges to its boards of managers. Those volunteer women certainly experienced their share of changes during the century and a half before they created the Poydras Home of today. And truth to tell, challenges remain as a third century of service begins.

But, patience: let us not speak yet of the present. Let us begin with a searching backwards glance into the deep past, when Louisiana was still French and Thomas Jefferson occupied the White House.

2

THE GENESIS OF AN IDEA

This is the man all tattered and torn
That kissed the maiden all forlorn
That milked the cow with the crumpled horn
That tossed the dog
That worried the cat
That chased the rat
That ate the malt
That lay in the house that Jack built.

In 1803, President Thomas Jefferson dispatched Robert Livingston and James Monroe to Paris to negotiate with the French for control of the strategically located city of New Orleans, thereby setting in motion a chain of events that led, ever so circuitously, to the eventual creation of the Poydras Asylum. To the world's amazement, Livingston and Monroe came away from their diplomatic foray with the entire Louisiana Territory, some 828,000 square miles of North America. When the whole of Louisiana fell into his lap, thus doubling the size of the United States, Jefferson moved briskly to secure funds from Congress to finance exploration of his surprise package. Although the names of William Dunbar and George Hunter do not vie for space in U.S. history books with those of the better-known Meriwether Lewis and William Clark, the unsung Dunbar and Hunter were the southern counterparts of that legendary pair of explorers.[1] Dunbar, of Natchez, more prominent and well-born than Hunter, was a friend of Thomas Jefferson. The president knew Hunter only by reputation, but that reputation persuaded Jefferson to enlist him. Jefferson wrote to Dunbar that Hunter's "fort[e] is chemistry, in that practical branch of science he has probably no equal in the

United States."[2] Hunter, born into a lower-middle-class family in Edinburgh and apprenticed to a druggist, had emigrated from Scotland at age nineteen, served as both an enlisted soldier and an apothecary in the Continental Army, and settled in Philadelphia after the Revolution. Like many an American with a modicum of scientific knowledge, Hunter soon began styling himself as "Doctor." He traveled extensively in the backcountry of Kentucky and Illinois, exploring, sampling minerals and water, and speculating in land, enjoying sufficient success as an explorer and scientist to provide a comfortable living for his growing family.

Requested by Jefferson to lead an expedition into the southwestern portion of the Louisiana Territory, co-leaders Dunbar and Hunter undertook to map the Ouachita River basin, collect data on minerals, water, flora, and fauna, and present a detailed report to the curious president. Beset by difficulties, Dunbar and Hunter got as far as "the hot springs" of present-day Arkansas by late 1804, but failed to complete their mission. Among various misadventures, Hunter's clumsy efforts to clean a firearm resulted in a gunshot wound that maimed two fingers and very nearly blew his thumb off. Powder burns caused temporary blindness, so that he, in agony and sightless for weeks, could not see to make entries in his journal. The consequences of his blunder acutely hampered Hunter's usefulness for most of the trip.

February 1805 found a recovering Hunter back in the relative comfort and safety of New Orleans, and no doubt relieved to be there. Partner Dunbar prepared to re-trace his steps and renew the mission, but the self-made Hunter, worried by the realization that his business interests had suffered seriously in his absence, chose to drop out and return to Philadelphia to attend to his wholesale drug firm. He was by this time past fifty years of age, and the rigors of another arduous river trip must have been daunting. Yet his unsuccessful exploration had accomplished one thing: George Hunter had met the city of New Orleans.

"This risk-saturated environment," as Lawrence Powell labeled it in his history of early New Orleans, had, in its first century of existence, already experienced floods, hurricanes, epidemics, and two particularly destructive citywide fires.[3] Though French in its first incarnation as a city in 1718, New Orleans and the Louisiana Territory had passed over to the Spanish crown in 1763 as part of the Seven Years' War settlement, but forty years later, Napoleon bullied the Spanish into ceding the land back to France. It was no sooner acquired than released, however, when Napoleon made his stunning bargain with Jefferson's envoys to sell *all* of Louisiana, collecting payment of just over $11 million from the Americans, pledging to cancel debts of nearly $4 million, and turning his focus to military conquest in Europe.

Exotic New Orleans differed profoundly from George Hunter's familiar Philadelphia. Eighty-five years of French and Spanish regimes had accustomed New Orleanians to autocracy such that leaders in Washington quite frankly distrusted the ability of locals to govern themselves according to the democratic principles of the fledgling United States. Indeed, rather than allow a territorial legislature of elected representatives for Louisiana, as precedent indicated, the distrustful federal government set up an appointive legislative council. A remarkably diverse population filled the city—French born and Spanish born, of course, but also arrivals from Francophone territories like Haiti and Canada; Anglo arrivals from the States, like Hunter himself; and a growing segment of "Creoles," a term used here to refer to native-born Louisianians, either of color or not, of French or Spanish heritage. Beyond the European elements, there were Choctaw, Natchez, Houmas, and other Native American tribes, in and around the city; there were enslaved Africans with roots in Senegambia, the Gold Coast, and Congo. Perhaps most unusual of all, one New Orleanian in five was a *gens de couleur libre,* a free person of color. And only one New Orleanian in five was an English speaker. "No city perhaps on the globe, in an equal number of human beings, presents a greater contrast of national manners, language, and complexion, than does New Orleans," observed a seemingly stunned Pennsylvanian, William Darby, in 1816.[4]

The New Orleans encountered by Hunter featured boisterous public dancing salons, where French and American patrons punctuated their disagreements over the band's choice of music with drawn swords, leading to scenes of frightened women fleeing pell-mell for safety. Governor William C. C. Claiborne had finally been forced to dispatch troops to maintain order amid the quadrilles. Illegal but wildly popular gambling houses proliferated, leading an American officer to observe, "Gambling in New Orleans is reduced to a profession."[5] A thirst for alcohol accompanied cards, dice, and games of chance; New Orleanians consumed prodigious quantities of liquors and wines, quite brazenly supplied by a robust smuggling trade. Depending upon point of view, the city might have been accurately described as rowdy and fun-loving, or lawless and hedonistic.

The Roman Catholic Church tried valiantly to tame this population. Capuchins, Jesuits, and Ursulines all toiled to minister to the spiritual and corporeal needs of residents, yet white Catholic men largely ignored their obligations (leading the archbishop to complain over their sparse attendance for Easter Communion, for example), meaning that the face of Catholicism in the city was primarily female and/or African. Among people of color, Voudou vied with Catholicism for primacy. Protestantism at the time of George Hunter's visit was represented in only a single fledgling congregation that had voted 45–7 to affiliate with the Episcopalians, the minority being seven Presbyterian votes; they met for a time in a boardinghouse on Bourbon Street. In short, organized religion countered hedonistic excess but feebly in early New Orleans. In the estimation of Hunter, a dour Scottish Presbyterian and a veteran of the American Revolution, the port city was almost wildly multicultural and untamed.

The decade 1805–1815 passed with the entrepreneurial Hunter engaged in business back in Philadelphia. His children grew to young adulthood. The year 1815 opened with news of the decisive though needless Battle of New Orleans, two weeks after the War of 1812 had officially ended. Materially aided by the Lafitte brothers and their Baratarian bandits, victorious general Andrew Jackson had also commanded backwoodsmen from Tennessee, free men of color, and Choctaw Indians in his rout of British forces. Wild celebrations followed in all U.S cities over this final smack to the former mother country. Though heavily French Louisiana had become a state only three years earlier and misgivings about the depth of her loyalty to the United States still nagged many Americans, now in the wake of such a stirring victory, Congress passed a resolution addressed "to the people of Louisiana and New Orleans." Unequivocally praising their "patriotism, fidelity, zeal and courage" as demonstrated during the battle, the resolution concluded emphatically that "the brave Louisianians deserve well of the whole people of the United States."[6]

Perhaps this ringing endorsement of the trustworthiness of exotic New Orleans caught Dr. George Hunter's notice, avowing as it did congressional faith in the transformation of erstwhile foreign New Orleanians into "true" Americans. At the same time, the city's population was surging; it topped 27,000 in the next census of 1820. Ships crowded the wharves, business boomed, and pathways to prosperity beckoned. Entrepreneurial Americans swarmed in from the northern states. One last time, George Hunter, the old opportunist, made his move; he determined to uproot his family and relocate to the cacophonous city on the Mississippi.

In 1815, Hunter, his wife Phoebe, and their five children, ranging in age from twelve to twenty-eight, crossed the Alleghenies in wagons and boated down the Mississippi River. The journal description of a twelve-year-old Quaker girl making the same crossing that year is representative of what the Hunters experienced. She reported: "We sometimes had to drive late to reach our destination. Then the wagons would seem to pitch from rock to rock and the descent was so steep that should we pitch over it would be hard telling where we should land."[7] The river leg of the journey required approximately three weeks, protracted because riverboatmen, rightly fearful of unseen impediments in the broad and swift waters, refused to run by night.

Once in New Orleans, the patriarch, assisted by his sons, established Hunter's Mills, which encompassed a rolling mill for sheet lead, iron, and copper, a mill for grinding barks and drugs, and a steam distillery. But Hunter's health soon failed; he seems to have suffered a form of dementia or possibly aphasia as the result of a stroke. When John James Audubon met the man he called "the renowned man of Jefferson," he noted sadly that Hunter was so diminished mentally that he could hardly communicate.[8] Dr. George Hunter lingered in this state for three more years, dying in his adopted city in 1823 and leaving a 63-year-old widow.

The wife who had accompanied her elderly but still adventurous husband to New Orleans was Phoebe Bryant Hunter (1760–1844), one of ten children of Thomas and Mary Shaw Bryant, devout Pennsylvania Quakers. Only two years old when her father died in Chester County, young Phoebe moved at age eleven with her mother and three sisters to Philadelphia. There the women were prompt to affiliate with the Society of Friends Southern District's Monthly Meeting, which proved an anchor of the familiar for the uprooted little Quaker family, newly arrived from rural realms into a strange and bustling city. The next fifteen years of being part of the Quaker community in Philadelphia, and, in particular, part of the separate women's business meetings, taught young Phoebe lessons of the heart and of the head, helping her to develop both compassion for the unfortunate and firm habits of system and order.

How or when Phoebe met her future husband is unknown, but it is certain that, in the eyes of her family, George Hunter's Presbyterian faith presented a serious impediment to their union. Though her widowed mother strongly attempted to dissuade her from marrying him, the 26-year-old Phoebe was mature enough to know her own mind. Two days after Christmas in 1786, understanding full well that marriage to Hunter would sever her bonds with the Society of Friends, Phoebe Bryant married her fiancé in the Second Presbyterian Church of Philadelphia, "having been cautioned and advised against it," according to minutes of the monthly meeting. The minutes further state that she married without her mother's consent "and contrary to the advice of friends."[9] Being accordingly read out of meeting, the headstrong Phoebe saw her ties to the church of her youth dissolved; she could no longer attend meeting, nor would her children be brought up within the Society of Friends. Phoebe Bryant Hunter was a Quaker no more.

Though she worshiped as a Presbyterian for the rest of her long life, Phoebe Hunter carried indelible lessons from her years among the Quakers. Philadelphia Quakeresses had practiced charity through their Friends' meetings since the late seventeenth century, but they significantly expanded their outreach efforts in the years just after the American Revolution. Historian Rosemary Abend argues persuasively that the Quakers' harsh experience as pacifist outcasts during the Revolution made them especially empathetic toward the sufferings of others.[10] In particular, young, unmarried Quaker women began to establish charitable associations in Philadelphia to minister to the multiple needs of the city's poor, most of whom had no margin for emergencies in their meager budgets. Illness or workplace injury could strike the laboring poor and bring temporary financial embarrassment, while permanently destitute individuals, especially the elderly, the disabled, and widows, were often frankly and tragically dependent upon charity for food, fuel, and other basic necessities. In the late eighteenth century, inspired by a female preacher and long accustomed to operating independently at sex-segregated Friends' business meetings, young Quaker women in Philadelphia established the Female Society for the Relief and Employment of the Poor (FSREP). The "relief" of their name involved distributing groceries, fuel, and clothing to the city's needy, especially during winter months, while "employment" meant offering paid work to poor women as spinners and seamstresses.

There was a decidedly gendered aspect to the Quaker women's benevolence; they felt keenly the distress of *women*. Acutely aware that women had few ways of earning, they gradually concentrated their efforts on helping poor women in any stage of life, but particularly elderly widows and young mothers with dependent children. With admirable logistical sense, the women of the FSREP divided Philadelphia into districts and assigned members to visit districts on a rotating basis, the better to identify and meet the needs of suffering and impoverished women. From repeated exposure to the woes of the urban poor, they gained "a practical understanding of the realities of working-class life, including the kinds of problems encountered by women attempting to support their families."[11] Seeing that women encumbered with small children could work only at home, these Philadelphia Quakers offered on-site childcare for women who worked in a community sewing room they had established. Recognizing that the duty of meal preparation ate away at women's hours for spinning and sewing, they began providing breakfast, dinner, and supper for the working women and their small children. They themselves worked long hours at their "House of Industry" each week, keeping accounts, filling and cleaning lamps, distributing flax, purchasing groceries, superintending the cooking, and laying the table properly for each meal. Every member of the benevolent association had her time-consuming turn at dispatching each of the requisite duties.

Phoebe Hunter, a wife and mother at the time of its 1795 founding, did not participate in Philadelphia's Female Society for the Relief and Employment of the Poor, composed as it was of unmarried women only. While the group seemed to have formulated no specific prohibition against the participation of wives, the labor-intensive realities of married women's lives in service to their own families devoured the hours they might have given to benevolent work in the community; records show only unmarried women working in FSREP. Phoebe Hunter, no longer a Quaker in good standing at this point, would not have been welcomed into a Friends' organization, regardless of her marital status. But her dechurched status did not require social shunning, and she surely maintained connections with her family, meaning that she must have talked with young relatives and girlhood friends who were part of the close circle of FSREP participants and from them, presumably, learned of FSREP activities.

The dire emergency of the 1793 yellow fever epidemic in Philadelphia brought Hunter out of her home and into the mainstream of benevolent work. She joined other Philadelphia women to distribute needed resources to homes where illness had wreaked havoc and distress. Out of the city's population of 45,000, perhaps 17,000 terrified citizens fled the contagion. Those Philadelphians who remained in town and kept their health shouldered the heavy burden of nursing thousands of desperately ill people. Phoebe Hunter helped care for victims, "ministering ... with her own hands to the relief and comfort of those suffering," according to her 1844 obituary.[12] During her years in Philadelphia, she was both a witness to and a part of what historian Bruce Dorsey has called "the pioneering forefront of voluntarism."[13] Beyond a doubt, the example of a well-organized women's benevolent association influenced Phoebe's thinking in later years in New Orleans.

After nearly thirty years of married life in Philadelphia, a series of chances combined to place Phoebe Hunter in the raw and bustling river port that some called "this great Sodom." After just over a year's residence in the Crescent City, the serene, plain-featured woman made a choice, the consequences of which ultimately affected thousands of lives. Moved by the plight of neglected and vulnerable girls whom she encountered near the markets and on the streets, convinced that they urgently needed a refuge, and conditioned by her years of Quaker voluntarism in Philadelphia, Phoebe Hunter convened a dozen like-minded women. Working together, they established the Female Orphan Society in New Orleans.

3

HUMBLE BEGINNINGS
AND A GENEROUS BENEFACTOR

One misty, moisty morning when cloudy was the weather,
I chanced to meet an old man, clothed all in leather.
He began to compliment, and I began to grin,
How do you do? And how do you do? And how do you do again?

When is an orphanage not really an orphanage? Perhaps when its existence is an unwelcome accident, which was the case in the spring of 1728 in the lower French Quarter of New Orleans. There, twelve recently arrived Ursuline nuns found themselves pursuing quite a variety of tasks in this rough and remote outpost of France: they pounded corn and rice, they scrubbed clothes, they taught the catechism, and they sheltered four orphaned girls in their convent. Operating an orphanage was only a sideline for the sisters, however; their preferred focus was emphatically female education, for both boarders and day students. The small stipend of 150 livres offered by the proprietary Company of the Indies for each orphaned girl in their care seems to have been the lure that led them to operate an asylum; the nuns needed this modest boost to their meager convent income. One year later, when Natchez Indians killed over two hundred men, women, and children upriver from New Orleans at Fort Rosalie, the kind sisters accepted thirty more endangered girls, survivors of the massacre. But as the number of their parentless charges increased so greatly, and the meager stipends provided for their care proved insufficient, the overworked nuns found themselves and their resources stretched thin; the influx of bereft, sickly, and often unruly children nearly overwhelmed the women. Without ever setting out to operate an orphanage, the compassionate Ursulines had stumbled into a situation that proved taxing and irritating. For the next ninety years, as their numbers of orphans waxed and waned, the sometimes reluctant sisters, while compiling a sterling record of successfully educating generations of girls and giving colonial Louisiana an unusually high rate of female literacy through their skillful teaching, continued to be, by default, the only institutional shelter for parentless children in the city. That changed, however, when the Female Orphan Society came into being in 1817.

The exact genesis of the Female Orphan Society in New Orleans is unclear; several versions of its birth have made their way into print over the decades since its establishment two centuries ago. In 1917, Daisy Hodgson, herself a board member of the society for more than four decades, alleged in a centennial remembrance of the Female Orphan Society that the arrival of twenty woebegone German children, orphaned by an epidemic raging on board their immigrant ship, led to the founding of her group. Tulane scholar John Smith Kendall, in a 1922 history of New Orleans, wrote that Mayor Augustin Macarty had urged Phoebe Hunter to spearhead an effort to provide care for indigent orphans. Kendall asserted, erroneously, that before this time New Orleans had not needed an orphanage. Seemingly unaware of the Ursulines' work, he implied that there had been no care at all provided for orphans prior to the Female Orphan Society's emergence and perpetuated the abiding story that the arrival of a fever-ridden immigrant ship debouching helpless orphans caused the unprecedented need for care. Lillian Fortier Zeringer, in her brief circa-1977 account of the history of the Poydras Home, did not further the German immigrant tale but noted that periodic epidemics created numbers of orphans in the city. Like Hodgson and Kendall, she placed Phoebe Bryant Hunter at the center of the group of women who established the Female Orphan Society. All agreed that, during 1816, Hunter and other women in her circle of friends took unfortunate children into their own homes for a short period before resolving to establish a residential shelter in their neighborhood.[1]

Over time, memories of the German immigrant ship and its cargo of misery quite naturally became cloudy, so that the perpetuated version of what led to the Poydras Asylum's founding turned out to be in error. In actuality, a Dutch ship loaded with German redemptioners experienced an outbreak of illness at sea, with death rates so high that several hundred souls, over half of those on board, died en route. When the wretched voyage finally ended and the ship docked in New Orleans, in March 1818, there were indeed orphans in need of care. However, the Female Orphan Society had been in existence for over one year at this time, so the plight of German orphan girls shivering on the docks assuredly did not serve as the catalyst for its formation. At the urging of Rev. Elias Cornelius, working in the city as an agent of the Connecticut Missionary Society, the managers of the Orphan Society did vote unanimously to give a home to the unfortunate children of the plague ship.

If not created in response to the plight of the German orphans, to what does the Poydras Asylum owe its start? In the early nineteenth century, newcomers from New England and eastern states exerted a significant influence on affairs in New Orleans, extending beyond commerce and politics. The city's Creole mayor Augustin Macarty knew George Hunter and his wife Phoebe well enough to appeal to them about the orphan situation, an indication that they had established themselves as people of prominence in less than two years' residence. This also hints that Mrs. Hunter, who famously had given heroic aid to the sick and suffering of Philadelphia during yellow fever epidemics there, had already become active in community benevolence in New Orleans. Yet paradoxically, although minutes of the first Female Orphan Society meeting of January 17, 1817, list nine women who served as the original officers and board of directors of the group (or "directresses," in the earliest usage), Phoebe Hunter's name is not among them.

In the group's minutes meticulously recorded over the next twenty-seven years, Phoebe Hunter shows up as a commanding presence, shaping policy and furthering the success of the institution, but she did not assume the formal role of "principal directress" until 1821. Perhaps modesty held her back; perhaps her household duties claimed her time; perhaps her husband objected or his deteriorating health prevented her. We have no way of knowing; however, subsequent generations of women who served as board members for the Female Orphan Society invariably cited Phoebe Hunter as the group's founding spirit. Indeed, years later, when she had recovered from a grave illness, the annual report for 1831 expressed the women's thankfulness that "a threatened calamity has been averted and the valued life of their beloved Directress been spared for further usefulness." Because of the esteem and veneration entertained for her character by other board members, they asked her to sit for a portrait to be placed in the boardroom adjacent to the likeness of benefactor Julien Poydras. "Modestly but firmly" Hunter declined, but the managers were not to be denied. After an interval of a few years, they sent a committee "to wait upon her" with the same request, and the 1837 minutes reported, "with much pleasure," that she acceded to their wish. Today, the portrait of Phoebe Bryant Hunter hangs in a place of honor in the Poydras Home, evidence of her leadership in the institution's first quarter century.[2]

The nine women identified as the organizers of the Female Orphan Society were recent arrivals to the newly American New Orleans, members of Protestant Anglo-American families with roots in the seaboard cities of the Northeast. The names recorded in the first minutes as original officers are Mrs. Hannah Nicholson and Mrs. N. K. Wolstoncraft, principal directors; Miss M. A. Hunter, secretary; Mrs. M. C. Morse, treasurer; and Mrs. A. Bryant, Mrs. A. H. Finley, Mrs. H. H. Brand, Mrs. A. M. Hennen, and Mrs. S. F. Morgan, directors.[3] Ties of consanguinity, class, and religion bound the founders together. M. A. Hunter was Mary Ann, Phoebe Hunter's thirty-year-old unmarried daughter, whose universally legible, firm handwriting and superb compositional skills recommended her for the secretary's position. Significantly, she elected to identify her fellow officers in minutes by the initials of their Christian names rather than those of their husbands. A. Bryant was Ann Bryant, Phoebe Bryant Hunter's sister-in-law. Hannah Nicholson, one of the two principal directors, was the mother of board member Ann Maria Hennen. Husbands of the women involved had attained prosperity as lawyers, commission merchants, businessmen, and politicians. Alfred Hennen and Nathan Morse achieved particular prominence: the former, born in Maryland and educated at Yale, was a veteran of the Battle of New Orleans and an esteemed Louisiana supreme court justice; the latter, born in New Jersey, was also a jurist and a politician who held the important municipal post of recorder in New Orleans. Morse was also a cousin of the inventor Samuel F. B. Morse.

Religion bound the Female Orphan Society founders most securely. The absence of Protestant congregations before the Louisiana Purchase had given the city a profoundly Catholic identity, even though many New Orleanians were but nominal Catholics at best. After 1803, migrants from the United States began arriving in numbers, bringing, in addition to their capital, their furnishings, and their families, a pronounced preference for Protestant worship. In 1805, Christ Church, the first Protestant congregation in New Orleans, took shape when the majority of newcomers voted to affiliate as Episcopalian. With the efforts of the newly arrived young Sylvester Larned, an enthusiastic Princeton-educated missionary, Presbyterianism was planted in the city in 1818. Only two years after the cornerstone was laid for Reverend Larned's church, however, the dreaded yellow fever claimed him as a victim. The twenty-four-year-old Larned had insisted on remaining in the city to minister to the sick during the summer epidemic, and he paid with his life. The real growth of Presbyterianism occurred under Larned's successor, the energetic and unconventional Theodore Clapp. In later life, Reverend Clapp characterized his early New Orleans congregation as consisting of "the ablest members of the Bar, those who had belonged to Congress, physicians, enlightened merchants, [and]... the conductors of the daily press."[4] His words describe male relatives of the founders and early supporters of the Female Orphan Society. When Clapp later abandoned strict Calvinism for the softer outlines of Unitarianism, some in his congregation followed right along, among them many of the leading Anglo-Saxon merchants of the city. The women who held leadership posts in the Female Orphan Society were represented in both Presbyterian and Unitarian congregations in the nineteenth century.

Early in 1817, having voluntarily given shelter to destitute orphan girls in their own homes for months, the founders of the Female Orphan Society moved to establish an organization, the timing of their activity leading one to suspect that perhaps a "new year's resolution" was involved. On January 10, 1817, they began soliciting female friends, who, by paying eight dollars, could become "subscribers" to underwrite the project, but would have no role in directing the organization. Energetic canvassing netted twelve hundred dollars from 150 women in one week's time. Nudging their acquaintances to remember that "the sum of two dollars four quarters [i.e., four times per year] is little more than one bitt [sic: bit, i.e., 12½ cents] per week," their dignified appeal observed that "even trifling exertions may be productive of much individual benefit" and insisted that such a negligible amount could "scarcely be missed by the giver." Their stated purpose in collecting these funds was to maintain and instruct indigent female orphans, with the ultimate goal of preparing them to support themselves in time. Forty-six gentlemen elected to assist the project. Declaring themselves "pleased with the late laudable exertions of the

Ladies of New Orleans," they too contributed the requisite eight dollars and became subscribers, "most joyfully." A few men gave larger donations, so that by the end of the week, the women had approximately $2,700 in hand.[5]

On January 17, 1817, a large number of female subscribers met to elect the society's officers, who, once chosen, were charged with writing a constitution for the body. In only four days they returned with a draft. The speed with which they produced this detailed framework for their orderly operation possibly signifies a borrowing from constitutions of other women's benevolent organizations. (This was not uncommon. For example, the practical Quaker Lucretia Mott had written her mother-in-law to ask for advice as she formed a group to relieve the poor, adding "if it is not asking too much, I should very much like to have a copy of your constitution.")[6] The New Orleans constitution revealed an expansion of the original mission, declaring the women's intent to provide a house "for the reception of indigent female orphans *and widows.*"[7] Over the years, the Female Orphan Society paid small stipends to poor widows in dire circumstances; by 1872, for example, they were providing very modest monthly pensions to seventy-five widows, and in the early years, they even offered living accommodations for a few widows in their asylum. However, the care of needy girls was always the society's predominant concern.

Evidently advised by individuals familiar with the law, the women promptly sought an act of incorporation from the state legislature, then in session in New Orleans, and were rewarded when that body passed the act in late February 1817. No doubt the connections of these women to men of standing in the community weighed heavily in their favor with the lawmakers. Here again, this move for incorporation indicates perhaps a familiarity on the part of the New Orleans Female Orphan Society with the actions of women's benevolent associations in other parts of the country. For example, in New York, the Female Society for the Relief of Poor Widows with Small Children had incorporated itself in 1802, as had the Female Orphan Society of Petersburg, Virginia, in 1812 and the Hartford Female Beneficent Society in 1813. Incorporation gave those women's groups distinct legal advantages, including rights that their members had lost upon marriage. In those days, the legal doctrine of coverture, transplanted into the United States from English common law, gave every husband almost unlimited power over his wife's property. Today we remember most vividly the fact that, upon marriage, a husband took absolute right to all of his wife's personal property, from the household goods and livestock that she brought to the union, to her jewelry and luxuries, down to and including the very clothing on her back. He owned any wages she might earn and controlled all real estate that was hers. Most significantly for women who formed benevolent associations with the idea of helping others, married women had no standing to make contracts, to sue, or to serve in the capacity of trustee, guardian, or administrator. They could not do business for themselves or others. The law summed it up bluntly by labeling them "civilly dead."

But in Louisiana, which abjured English common law in favor of a hybrid code based on French and Spanish law, married women enjoyed a different, somewhat less diminished status. They could retain ownership of both the personal and the real property that they owned at the time of marriage and enjoy full right to all that they earned as wives.[8] Often remarked upon is the fact that a Louisiana wife was entitled to half of all a couple's community assets in case of divorce, plus all her separate property. However, other clauses in the code darkened this rosy scenario considerably. Although not laboring under the burdens of coverture, Louisiana wives were nonetheless forbidden to "alienate, grant, mortgage, or acquire" property without husbands' explicit written permission. They were further barred from appearing in court for any reason without their husbands' consent. If allowed to stand, these considerable disabilities would effectively prevent the Female Orphan Society from operating, since who in the business world would ever make contracts with these women if the contracts could not be enforced in a court of law?[9]

An act of incorporation thus became an essential part of the women's apparatus for success because it awarded their group the right to sue and defend itself in court, to make contracts, to accept bequests, and, crucially, to own, buy, and sell real estate. Corporate status cleverly allowed Phoebe Hunter and her married friends to circumvent their own diminished legal position through the creation of the Female Orphan Society, a body that had legal rights but possessed no sex. The act passed by the Louisiana legislature and copied verbatim into the group's minutes enumerated the rights awarded thereby to the women's group, stating that they could now exercise these rights "as fully as *any natural person.*"[10]

Gaining this incorporated status paved the way for the women of the Female Orphan Society to press the limits of gender propriety. The significance of their undertaking should not be underestimated. They would now have legal standing to raise and manage money, to spend and invest as they saw fit, to buy property, to hire and dismiss employees, and to deal with city and state government, *all without male control*. From our twenty-first-century vantage point, the work of women to shelter orphaned girls seems unremarkable, but for their times, these women were stepping far beyond their appointed sphere, the home, and inserting themselves into public space, which had hitherto been exclusively male space. Their incorporation made them a group of women perfectly at liberty to seek male advice, but equally at liberty to disregard it.

The women quickly assigned some of their number to identify "suitable objects" for their charity, while others took the task of locating an appropriate house to rent. Only three weeks after they had begun their subscription drive, Female Orphan Society secretary Mary Ann Hunter recorded momentous news in her minutes: the society had received a munificent donation, a large lot with a house that could serve as their asylum![11] The gift of this spacious old plantation house, ideally located at the corner of St. Charles Avenue and Julia Street in Faubourg St. Mary, the American sector of the city where the managers of the Female Orphan Society resided, would serve their purposes well. Here is the first example of what would become a motif of most timely good fortune, a motif that, as this narrative will reveal, has run like a bright red thread through the tapestry of two centuries of Poydras history.

The grateful Female Orphan Society immediately voted that its asylum should bear the name of the generous citizen whose unexpected largesse had so delighted them. Writing to this kindly patron, secretary Hunter assured him that "the prayers of the fatherless and the widow, never offered in vain, shall ascend to the Most High for blessings on his head" and predicted that angels would observe his gift with joy while all heaven itself took note. In her rapturous vision of celestial approval, Hunter foresaw his name engraved on tablets "more durable than marble." Whether these remarkable events trans-pired in the cosmos remains unknown, but it is certain that the last part of her letter came to pass; she mused presciently that "children, yet unborn" would repeat his name "with thanksgiving and praise."[12]

The life of this benefactor, Julien Poydras, embodied a rags-to-riches motif in most tellings.[13] Born in Nantes in 1746, and a veteran of early adventures as a captured cabin boy pressed into service in the British navy, the young

Frenchman soon stowed away to Santo Domingo and, from the Caribbean island, made his way to New Orleans in 1768. Conflicting accounts exist regarding his financial condition upon arrival; most call him penniless, but some maintain that he came from an affluent family of French merchants and could hardly have arrived without some wherewithal. All agree that young Poydras was for a time an itinerant carrying a pack, peddling pots, knives, and trinkets to the settlers of Pointe Coupée Parish, some 110 miles upriver from New Orleans. Through his industry, he prospered sufficiently to buy land and open a modest store in the settlement there. Steadily he built the store into a thriving mercantile warehouse that supplied scattered communities throughout the lower Mississippi Valley with fabric, tools, medicines, groceries, and spirits. He owned the boats that shipped his goods, and like most merchants of that time, he functioned as lender, extending credit and making cash loans. Little by little he amassed land, sometimes receiving Spanish land grants during the time of Spain's possession of Louisiana, and more often purchasing and then consolidating likely plots. Ultimately, Julien Poydras owned seven rich Louisiana plantations and upwards of five hundred slaves. This huge force of human property—men, women, and children who worked his cotton, cane, and indigo crops; tended his cattle; and operated his cotton gins and press—meant that the former pack peddler, who once carried all his merchandise on his back, by the early nineteenth century ranked as one of the largest slaveholders in antebellum America.

Since there were many ways of practicing slave ownership, we might pause here to inquire what sort of slave owner Julien Poydras was. Significantly, the 1795 Pointe Coupée slave revolt, the most massive uprising among the enslaved in America to that date, was plotted on the estate of Poydras. The seeds of the uprising were sown well in advance. Some of Poydras's slaves, accused of plotting an earlier revolt, served time in a jail in New Orleans and were put to work unloading ships there. On the docks, they mingled with "Louisiana's multinational, multiracial underclass of deported convict laborers and soldiers whose character and social class differed little from the rejects and deserters sent to Louisiana under French rule."[14] This association exposed them to a turbulent stew of news and ideas, based on events in blood-soaked France, meaning that when these particular slaves were released to return to Pointe Coupée, they took with them the heady ideology of the French Revolution and the news that France's revolutionary government had voted to abolish slavery.

Antoine Sarrasin, the *commandeur,* or Creole overseer, on Poydras's estate, led the conspiracy. Later testimony indicated that many Poydras slaves were involved in the plot, as were many from surrounding estates. They planned to start a fire in a cabin on the Poydras plantation and then kill whites who ran to fight the blaze. After arming themselves with weapons and ammunition from the immense stock kept in the Poydras warehouse, they intended to rampage through the countryside, killing and liberating as they went. Whites detected the plot a few days after Easter 1795, and Spanish colonial administrators moved swiftly to mete out harsh justice. In June, twenty-three slaves were hanged and then beheaded. Grimly determined authorities took an added step: they nailed the severed heads onto posts all along the roadway leading from Pointe Coupée to New Orleans in a grisly display meant to deter future resistance. In a letter to his kinsman, Poydras observed tersely, "They hung 20,000 piasters worth of my negroes."[15]

Was discontent greater on the estate of Julien Poydras than on other Louisiana plantations? Certainly, the Poydras estate had a most atypical slave population, one that featured a drastic sex imbalance, and this was by the owner's design. Whereas on most plantations, a rough parity between the sexes had developed by the early nineteenth century, on the Poydras estate adult men outnumbered women of childbearing age by more than ten to one. In consequence, the men Poydras enslaved were forced to find sex partners on other plantations, forfeiting the comforts of family and domesticity, and, as a result, were certainly discontented and resentful of the situation. Historian Gwendolyn Midlo Hall speculates that "Poydras did not like young women, especially young Creole women." Moreover, Poydras often purchased very young children without their mothers, perhaps because he intended to teach them habits and patterns without interference from parents—"to mold his slave force to his liking," as Hall puts it. In 1786, he purchased a four-year-old boy and a seven-year-old girl in exchange for a strapping young adult male, plus a payment of 100 piasters. When he learned that little Honore suffered from epilepsy, however, he filed suit against the seller in order to negate the deal.[16] Squaring this cold, calculating planter with the kindly old gentleman held in fond memory by generations of Poydras Home orphans is indeed an exercise in cognitive dissonance, as is the realization that the philanthropic rescue of countless needy or neglected girls rested on a fortune produced by enslaved workers.

Julien Poydras the merchant-planter-slaveholder had urban and political interests as well. Less than ten years after his modest start as a peddler, he purchased a Bourbon Street residence in New Orleans.[17] Over time, he acquired lots on the city's main thoroughfares (Dumaine, Chartres, St. Ann, Burgundy, and the eponymous Poydras) as well as along the busy riverfront. Increasingly, he divided his time between the planter's life in Pointe Coupée and his new role in the territorial capital of New Orleans, where he took a leading part in the government of Louisiana.

After the 1803 transfer of Louisiana from France to the United States, American officials had ample reason to doubt the loyalty of the French-speaking locals, who had previously resisted the Spanish takeover of their colony with violence in New Orleans; Americans feared they would be no more supportive of the new arrangement with the United States. Thus it was with great relief that they learned about Julien Poydras, an outspoken backer of the U.S. regime, whose fluency in English and noted probity of character recommended him highly to the Americans. W. C. C. Claiborne and James Wilkinson, the first governors of Louisiana, wrote President Thomas Jefferson in praise of Poydras only months after the transfer. Accordingly, Jefferson appointed Poydras to a seat on the legislative council for the Territory of Orleans, and that body promptly elected Poydras its president. When the territory became eligible for statehood, Poydras energetically championed the wisdom of welcoming Louisiana into the United States and successfully persuaded dubious federal lawmakers, one of whom had memorably voiced his reluctance to admit "the heathens of that swamp country" into the Union. The 1811 passage of the enabling act gave Louisiana the right to write a constitution, elect a governing body, and choose delegates to Congress. Once again, Poydras was the choice of his peers, this time to preside over the state convention at which these details were accomplished. When the Louisiana state government was organized, Poydras emerged as president of the state senate, a post he held intermittently until his death.

Despite Julien Poydras's roles as planter, slaveholder, merchant, and statesman, education and charitable giving constitute his most lasting legacies. Primarily self-taught, Poydras possessed the autodidact's high regard for formal education. He lived an unostentatious life on his simply furnished main plantation, with few luxuries, but he did allow himself the indulgence of books and prized his expensive library of more than five hundred volumes. Once he grasped the levers of political power in Louisiana, Poydras used them to press for free public schools. It gave him pleasure that his home district of Pointe Coupée led the way, establishing five free schools in 1808, no doubt with his special encouragement. He donated land for one school and served as first president of his parish's school board.

A distinct air of eccentricity clings to Julien Poydras. Alcée Fortier, writing in 1903, described him as a man of the eighteenth century who dressed as if still living in the era of Louis XV, 1710–1774. An inventory of his personal goods taken at the time of his 1824 death counted three snuff boxes, seventeen pairs of knee breeches (though he also possessed long trousers), and 136 pairs of stockings, all hallmarks of a much earlier time. This wealthy man who dressed in such antiquated style never married. Melodramatic stories of a lost love circulated, although without a scintilla of supporting evidence. Rich, politically powerful, esteemed by his peers, but without the comforts of consort or children, Poydras late in life turned his attention to providing for two classes of unfortunate females: poor girls without dowries and female orphans. His will provided $30,000 for dowries of young women in his home parish, stipulating that preference would go to those in pitiable circumstances. He evidently saw the burdens of indigent females as being exceedingly great, given the demands of gender propriety and the difficulties unattached girls would have in making their way alone in the world; his concern for helping poor girls to make successful marriages is proof of that.[18]

In a lengthy address to the legislative council in New Orleans in 1809, Poydras employed a memorable figure of speech, calling the Territory of Orleans "an adopted child in a great family." Although Poydras himself had created no family, great or otherwise, having (presumably) sired no children to carry his name, in old age his thoughts turned to the plight of female children without parents. When the women of the Female Orphan Society canvassed for subscriptions, Poydras promptly contributed $100. Less than a month later, after the women had boldly approached him to request that he increase his gift, he startled the group by offering them the use of his New Orleans plantation house, a large structure of distinctly West Indian aspect.

The Female Orphan Society took possession of the house at Julia and St. Charles in late February 1817 and set to work readying it to serve as their orphanage. In their own homes, these women provided clothing, nourishment, and safety for their biological children. They would endeavor to do the same for orphaned girls and a few indigent widows at Poydras, by making a donated building into a livable, functional home. As wives and mothers, well accustomed to managing the smooth operation of homes, they turned with confidence to the task of buying necessary items for the asylum: mosquito netting and mattresses, coarse material for towels, a tin-plate stove, a barrel of sugar. Because they knew the contents and workings of a well-ordered residence, this part of their task must have seemed quite familiar.

By early March 1817, the women announced in a notice in the *New Orleans Gazette* that the Poydras Asylum was ready to receive "all such objects as are embraced by their constitution ... indigent widows and female children, particularly orphans,"[19] to whom it would offer a home, food, clothing, education, and medical care if needed. One notes that they advertised shelter for female children, particularly *but not exclusively* orphans. They recognized that the exigencies of life did not allow some parents to provide adequately for their children. Furthermore, the absolute inadequacy of any kind of poor relief in New Orleans had harsh consequences for the young.

Thus, from the outset, the home prepared to accept full orphans, half orphans, and girls whose living parents manifestly could not care for them. Of those admitted in the first seven years, 32 percent were full orphans, but 63 percent had one parent living, meaning that the institution, like many others, was, from the start, less an orphanage and more a residential childcare center serving the deserving poor. The half orphans on average lived in the asylum for not quite six months before being claimed by a parent, almost always a mother.[20] Obviously, the surviving parent used the asylum as temporary shelter in time of distress.

The female founders of Poydras never intended to assume the quotidian operation of the asylum themselves; employing a residential staff, they would give intelligent supervision as the home's board of managers. Initially, in addition to laboring women for kitchen and laundry duties, they chose to hire a factotum they styled as "governess," whose duties far outdistanced the merely pedagogical and encompassed physical and moral responsibilities as well. The governess, according to rules the women promulgated, would have the girls "up, washed, combed, and dressed at sunrise," would conduct morning devotions with them before breakfast, and would then teach them in the school-room until noon and again after midday dinner until five o'clock. Sundays had a specific rhythm, for the governess would accompany them to church, taking care that all behaved with decorum and reverence. Once back at the asylum, she would provide an hour of religious instruction, emphasizing to the girls "the presence of God, His perfection, His hatred of sin, His love of holiness, and their own accountableness to Him for all actions." In the early months, first a Mrs. Taylor, then a Mrs. Hohlheim, then a Mrs. Titley tried and failed to satisfy the demands of the position. The board members turned to Rev. Sylvester Larned for help in locating a suitable person, stipulating in a letter to him that she must be "a woman of strict piety, who will devote her attention entirely to the care of the asylum, who will *consider the family as her adopted children,* who will regulate their time and actions, and show by her example still more than by precept that she is indeed anxious to lead them to religion and virtue." At last, with the minister's assistance, they settled on Miss Mary Clark, who came to them from Philadelphia and proved to be highly satisfactory.[21]

The nineteenth century took gender differences very seriously. Middle-class women claimed greater moral virtue than men and found this claim universally acknowledged. Working from this premise, women felt that they had a duty to teach virtue to others, to uplift, cleanse, and purify, through words and example. The women of Poydras firmly intended to give the girls in their care not only physical but also moral protection from the outside world. Just as they carefully guarded the morals of their own daughters and instructed them by word and example in proper conduct, so they planned to mold the orphans into virtuous beings, as indicated in their detailed instructions to Reverend Larned regarding the qualities they sought in a governess.

Summarizing the disabilities peculiar to orphaned girls, historian Suzanne Lebsock aptly labeled them "sexually endangered, intellectually disadvantaged, and economically vulnerable."[22] In the view of the Female Orphan Society founders, their vulnerable charges needed the double shield of a solid education and a sound moral character to keep them from want and misery. In the managers' estimation, the most troubling possible consequence of a poor upbringing was the likelihood that, devoid of the necessary foundation provided by education and good character, a girl would stray into a depraved, degraded life of vice. Contemplation of this distressing outcome appears to have animated the founding mothers of the Poydras Asylum. The society's first annual report, penned by Mary Ann Hunter, hints obliquely at the dangers from which "the family" needed protection. Expressing the managers' surprise over the number of people in New Orleans who were in "absolute want," even though living "in a country whose industry has so many inducements to labor," the young secretary traced the cause to "an improper education."[23] In this passage, Hunter, articulating thoughts presumably shared by the Poydras board of managers, was explicitly stating her negative reaction to the great numbers of refugees from Santo Domingo and Cuba who had by this date become a very visible component of the population of New Orleans.

Beginning in 1793, displaced French colonials fleeing the Haitian revolution in Santo Domingo had streamed away from that chaotic island, sometimes accompanied by their slaves. Often, they settled in Cuba. However, in 1809, as a result of war between Spain and France, Spanish-governed Cuba expelled all Santo Domingan refugees who would not swear allegiance to Spain, a policy that caused an enormous wave of French-speaking refugees to flood into Francophone New Orleans. When more than ten thousand newcomers arrived in less than one year, they doubled the city's population and precipitated a crisis as the city struggled to provide temporary relief. The French community in New Orleans responded sympathetically, but not so the already outnumbered American element, which resented this reinforcement of the French-speaking majority. When Mary Ann Hunter generalized in her minutes that people "in absolute want" were "generally fugitives from the islands of St. Domingo and Cuba who have been accustomed to no exertion but that of commanding," she was expressing the bias of her Anglo-American class. Hunter and the other managers of the Female Orphan Society hailed from ethnically homogeneous eastern states, and like the white merchants and professionals who were their fathers and husbands, they were, in the words of historian Paul LaChance, "unwilling to adjust to the cosmopolitan character of New Orleans society." Upon arrival from her native Philadelphia just over two years before, Hunter had voiced her blunt reaction: "what a strikingly ugly and wretched city to experience," she wrote to her cousin Eliza, adding that she found the "language of the people" was "very grating to [her] ears."[24]

The influx of Santo Domingan refugees consisted of three groups: white

Europeans, enslaved Africans, and free people of color. Among the free people of color who fled to New Orleans from Haiti, women outnumbered men by more than three to one, whereas, among white refugees, there were twice as many men as women. With such an imbalance between the sexes, following a long-established pattern from the Caribbean that was by no means unknown in New Orleans, no doubt some of the white men entered openly into domestic partnerships with women of color, though the law forbade their marriage. Such miscegenous unions would have been distasteful to the Anglo Protestant women of the Female Orphan Society, as would any men's liaisons with prostitutes. The city's mayor commented upon the presence of many destitute young women among the white element of island fugitives as well. Presumably, these were the women whom Hunter had in mind when she wrote disapprovingly in her first annual report to the Female Orphan Society, commenting on their low condition: "miserable and helpless, incapable of either mental or corporeal activity ... yielding to the temptations of vice to procure a momentary suspension of their wretchedness, not reflecting that they are adding guilt to poverty, and thus becoming wretched indeed."[25]

If the "vice" exhibited by some of the impoverished young refugee women from Santo Domingo was the exchange of sex for money in order to live, the managers of the Female Orphan Society would have found that conduct reprehensible. Over seven hundred white women and perhaps another three hundred white female children had arrived in New Orleans with the refugee tide. If some of them "yield[ed] to the temptations of vice," as Hunter alleged, they presented a damaging, demoralizing example for a younger generation of females. Hunter's 1818 annual report stated that the managers chose to focus their efforts on saving unprotected girls from future vice, rather than on redeeming so-called "fallen women" from present transgression. In order to prevent future misery, they made their mission "the maintenance and education of unprotected children of their own sex" and expressed their aim "to rescue from want, and in most cases infamy, those unfortunate children who are thrown upon the world without protection."[26] Clearly, the asylum was a response to perceived immorality and disorder.

Beyond encasing their orphans in a protective carapace of morality, the founders intended to provide the girls with a solid education "in all useful knowledge and labor whereby they may earn a support for themselves," ob-

serving pointedly that "charity is never so well bestowed as when it is employed in qualifying its objects to live independently of its bounty."[27] The
curriculum offered in the Poydras schoolroom included mornings devoted to
reading, writing, spelling, arithmetic, practical needlework, and religious studies. It featured none of the "ornamentals" such as music, drawing, modern lan-
guages, or fancy needlework that so often graced the antebellum educations
of girls from the comfortable classes. In the afternoons, Poydras girls learned
domestic skills such as cooking, cleaning, washing, ironing, and sewing. Education and moral training at the Poydras Asylum aimed to equip a young
woman to move into adulthood prepared to be an upstanding, pious, and
competent wife and mother in a modest home of her own, or a respectable,
self-supporting single woman should an offer of marriage not be forthcoming.

Ironically, indigent girls residing at the Poydras Asylum received a better
education than virtually any girls of average means in the entire city of New
Orleans. Daughters of the comfortable classes might study privately with tu-
tors and governesses or be educated by the Ursulines, but options for the mid-
dling classes were few indeed. For decades, there were no public schools for
girls. When they were established, a requirement that parents declare themselves indigent in order to enroll their daughters was part of the deal. Since
upstanding citizens of modest means quite naturally recoiled from the stigma
of labeling themselves paupers for the sake of educating their girls, Poydras
girls in the early years acquired an education that few other New Orleans
daughters of working parents obtained.

Initially, the Poydras managers planned to educate their charges using the
Lancastrian system, a monitorial approach in which the more advanced students taught the less advanced ones. Joseph Lancaster, the English Quaker
who designed the eponymous plan, had toured the United States in the early
nineteenth century, lecturing on his pedagogical methods, and shortly after
the Poydras Asylum opened its doors in New Orleans, Philadelphia had established a school for training teachers in the Lancastrian system. The Lancastrian method had the virtue of being an inexpensive way to educate numbers
of children, and it was certainly in vogue for educating poor children at the
time of the Female Orphan Asylum's founding. No doubt, the Philadelphia
and Quaker connections of some Poydras managers influenced the founders
to consider Lancaster's way, but, in the end, they wisely elected to hire a com-

petent teacher and even to pay for an assistant in her classroom, rather than to consign their little charges to instruction from other orphans only a bit more advanced than they.

The minutes of the Poydras board of managers' meetings contain evidence of the early officers' compassion and gentleness. In March 1818, the Rev. Elias Cornelius encountered the just-arrived German orphans shivering on the wharf, having barely survived a nightmarish voyage during which disease claimed hundreds of lives. He recalled that their pitiful condition moved him greatly: "One was a sickly looking infant of two years of age. Another was four years old, with but one tattered garment, and that so poor that I was compelled to tie my handkerchief about its body, to hide its nakedness. Some of them were laboring under the worst cutaneous diseases, others were almost covered with vermin, and all were extremely filthy."[28]

Reverend Cornelius went directly to the managers of the Female Orphan Asylum, an indication that, after little more than a year of existence, their organization had established a reputation for benevolence. They were, providentially, holding their weekly board meeting at that very hour. He recorded that his account of the sick children, suddenly bereft of parents and utterly without protection in a foreign city, literally moved the women to weep. After their tears, however, they sprang into action. The minister marveled that within only a few hours, he had the pleasure of seeing the little waifs "washed, fed, and neatly clad," by the intervention of Poydras managers. Two older girls had sailed as indentured servants. Before being allowed to take them into their care, the women paid $160 to redeem their contracts. By the end of the day, the asylum was home to seven German girls.[29]

Even in its earliest and leanest years of operation, the Poydras Asylum never fit the cheerless Dickensian stereotype of a grim, austere building staffed by crabbed disciplinarians who doled out thin soup and scriptures to pitiful little waifs. When the managers spoke of "the home" and "our family," there seems to be no reason to doubt their sincerity. Recognizing that the orphans in their care deserved to have their childish wants gratified on occasion, they provided indulgences as well as necessities; for example, early records show expenditures for candy as well as for soap. To recognize good work and good conduct, they provided modest prizes. In April 1822, the minutes note their decisions: "Betsy Calava shall have reward for reading, Doxy for sewing,

Susan for spelling, Patsy for writing, Mary Lamasny for gentleness and obedience."[30] The managers borrowed the concept of offering concrete rewards
for good performance from the Lancastrian system of education. Early practitioners of the psychological principle of positive reinforcement, they awarded
new gloves and silver thimbles to girls who were eager to please and so sought
to mold the character and behavior of their young charges.

"Lady managers" visited the asylum regularly to observe its operation and
learn its needs. Sharing meals with the girls led them to take care with menus
to provide nutritious and tolerably appetizing fare. The routine offerings were
simple and frugal, and quantity no doubt varied, but the menu was not spartan. Breakfast in the early years consisted of wheat bread or cornbread and
butter, with steaming café au lait or glasses of milk. The main meal, midday
dinner, varied according to day. On Monday, Wednesday, and Saturday, the
girls were served soup with boiled meat and hominy or rice. On Tuesday and
Thursday, they ate gumbo with meat and rice or hominy. Friday brought fish,
and Sunday's big dinner consisted of roast meat with vegetables and bread.
Dessert meant boiled or baked puddings. Suppers were simple—either corn
mush or rice with molasses, or tea with bread and butter.[31]

The task of governing admissions thrust each manager into an early social worker's role. Managers sought to learn the circumstances of every child
who was brought to them by seemingly well-meaning strangers or distraught
mothers or fathers. When an adult requested a child's admission, the board
typically appointed two managers to learn more about the situation and then
heard their recommendations at the next meeting. A routine entry in the minutes reads as follows: "Madame Lemoine for the admission of a poor girl. Mrs.
Kennedy & Mrs. Duplessis named to wait upon her to enquire into the circumstances." Petitions from concerned citizens flowed steadily to the women
asking for the admission of needy girls. "One from Mr. Berry requesting the
admission of a German child. One from Judge Workman requesting entrance
for the child of a distressed widow." Sometimes there was urgency to an admission request, as in the plea of a very poor woman who had "married a
Spaniard who ill-treated her child so dreadfully that its life was in danger."[32]

The Poydras managers also regulated withdrawals from the institution.
They usually allowed surviving parents to reclaim their children when their
circumstances improved. However, they were frankly loath to release girls if,

in their judgment, home conditions remained chaotic or endangering; their confidence that the asylum's well-regulated environment was sometimes the better option was unshakeable. Accordingly, they began to require that, as a prerequisite for admission, girls be bound to the board for a term, usually until they reached the age of sixteen. Typically, an indigent parent surrendered her parental rights when she surrendered her child by signing an instrument transferring custody. With this power, the managers might, but were not required to, release a girl when a surviving parent appealed for her; all rested with their judgment and not the parent's desire.[33]

Having a legal hold on the girls of their institution opened the door for managers themselves to bind older girls out to responsible adults who met their approval. The managers' guidelines mandated that persons taking children must sign articles vowing to teach them a trade or skill, or provide a cash payment at the end of their term of service. In the first fifteen years of operation, the managers bound out some 20 percent of the girls to families; after thirty-five years, 12 percent of Poydras girls had been apprenticed. Girls so apprenticed were usually eleven years of age or older. Binding out steadily declined with the passage of time.

Seemingly exercising caution and due diligence about indenturing the Poydras girls, the managers sifted through applications from the community for their labor. Minutes indicate their firm belief that gaining an education outweighed all other factors for the girls in their charge. In 1827, a Mrs. Carroll applied for six girl apprentices whom she wished to teach the trade of mantua making. The managers assented "with eagerness" to send four, but, although there were ninety-nine girls then in residence, they replied that they "regret they cannot at this moment send the number she requested," an indication that they felt no others were sufficiently advanced to be removed from the schoolroom. In the annual report for 1846, the secretary recorded a total population of 142, with seventy admissions and thirty girls placed in "suitable homes," while also noting the rejection of "numerous" applications for girls because managers "prefer[ed] to retain them longer in the school." They avoided placing girls in situations where they would primarily be nursemaids to young children, believing it was important to position them where they would learn skills such as millinery, dressmaking, or, at the very least, the broad array of domestic arts necessary to household management.[34]

The system of "binding out" depended upon the diligence of managers, who either had personal knowledge, or made it their business to gain knowledge, of the adults who stepped forward to apply for girls. They interviewed applicants and visited their homes. The managers unhesitatingly judged the character of adults who applied and rejected those who fell short of an unstated but seemingly understood standard of morality. "Mrs. Downey requested to have one bound to her," the minutes noted vaguely in 1823. "It is not thought proper to consent."[35] They consulted the girls themselves, and it appears that compulsory apprenticeships were most uncommon at the asylum. A committee regularly visited the apprenticed girls to observe their living conditions and degree of satisfaction; they removed children from situations they deemed inappropriate. Often, they allowed applicants to take girls "on trial" for one or two months and then interviewed the young apprentices in an attempt to assess the situation. Finally, they made every effort to place Catholic girls with Catholic families, and Protestant with Protestant, trying to ensure the best experience possible for each girl.

Records indicate that managers were canny enough to know that appearances could be deceiving. When Mrs. Southmayd made a home visit to check on conditions, she found the place "looking neat & comfortable & saw nothing to disapprove," but a concerned neighbor informed her that all was not well with Rebecca, the young apprentice sent from Poydras. Since a wary Rebecca would not complain in the presence of her employer, the manager prudently took her back to the asylum, where she testified to her unhappiness ("she is not well treated, has to work very hard, never goes to church and seldom goes to school"). She was returned to the asylum.[36]

The managers were not above violating their policies when it was expedient. For example, they responded to their teachers' frequent complaints about young Ann Johnston's behavior by determining to place her out with a woman who needed a caregiver for her child. In this case, ridding the asylum of a disruptive troublemaker and a bad influence on the group carried more importance than ensuring one individual girl's education and acquisition of worthwhile skills. Nevertheless, they stipulated that the arrangement was for one month on trial and that in no way should this action "be considered a precedent for the future disposal of the orphans." (Over four years later, when managers learned that the apprenticed Ann Johnston was to be married, clearly not feeling unkindly toward her, they voted to provide her with an appropriate trousseau.)[37]

The practice of binding out declined rapidly after the Civil War and had virtually melted away by the 1870s, but in the asylum's early years, binding out could frequently be a successful strategy. By apprenticing girls, practical Poydras managers aimed to pair children who needed stable homes with responsible community members whose households needed labor, in the process freeing space at the asylum for younger, less sturdy, more vulnerable girls. Ruth W. Herndon and John E. Murray, scholars of the apprentice system in early America, have judged that, as a rule, apprenticing "was neither success nor failure but rather a holding pattern. It kept vulnerable children alive, it put them in a family setting, it put them to work at some useful occupation, and it familiarized them with the kind of manual labor that was the lot of most early Americans."[38]

Early on, the managers suspected that unscrupulous or irresponsible adults were not above taking advantage of the charity their institution extended to needy girls. They feared that some parents who actually had the means to pay for their daughters' care at Poydras merely used the institution when they found it inconvenient to dispatch their parental obligations, retrieving their children when they were inclined to do so. At the women's request, the state legislature in 1819 passed a bill prohibiting the removal of any child from the asylum, even by a parent, without managers' approval, "except a remuneration for the maintenance of such child should be made to the Society." It stated that "whenever any child the object of indigence or wretchedness has been duly received into the asylum ... it shall not be lawful for the relations ... to take the said child without the consent ... of the directors of said asylum, unless the relations pay the amount which shall be determined by arbitrators of the expenses incurred by the asylum from the time the child was admitted in it." Armed with this law, the managers could, at their discretion, collect payment from parents who had left their children with the asylum while they traveled, conducted business, or dealt with a crisis. In particular, their energies in the early years seem to have been turned on former refugees who were returning to Cuba. When Caroline Ferdinand's father wrote that he wished her sent to him at "Havanna," they observed in the minutes that "from the representation of his situation, it appeared that he was well able to afford one hundred dollars per annum for the time she had been there."[39] He subsequently paid and claimed Caroline.

Racial practices dictated that the asylum would receive only white females. The managers had no hesitation about admitting children of Latin parentage, but they took pains to ascertain that such girls were not of mixed race. After manager Celeste Duplessis secured admission of "a little Spanish child" in 1836, she, evidently pressed by the other managers, provided a certificate of baptism for Maria, which they placed among the asylum's important papers. The secretary bluntly explained their reasoning: "This little unfortunate was so extremely dark complexioned that the Managers were anxious to secure for it, this respectable proof of its *white* parentage."[40]

The question of finances routinely occupied the Female Orphan Society managers in the early years. They had opened their doors to needy girls when they had but little in their purse, firm in the belief that more would be found for this humanitarian work. The clergy proved to be one source of funds. Several local ministers preached charity sermons and donated their collections to the Female Orphan Society. Of particular note, indicating a degree of Protestant-Catholic cooperation in this endeavor, is the fact that Father Antonio de Sedella, the celebrated Père Antoine of St. Louis Cathedral, allowed a Baptist missionary from Georgia to speak in his church to raise money for the asylum. On that occasion, the ecumenical visitor spoke in French, and Catholic worshippers contributed sixty dollars. That afternoon, the Georgian repeated his message in English, to the Protestants at Christ Church, and netted ninety-five dollars for the asylum. Female Orphan Society minutes remarked on the managers' gratitude to Pere Antoine "for the unprecedented favor of permitting a Protestant minister to officiate in his church."[41]

Far more lucrative than the clerical connection was the managers' relationship with state and local governments, ties cultivated from the first month of their existence. One of the original managers of the Female Orphan Society was Martha Nicholls Morse, wife of city councilman Nathan Morse, a happy circumstance for the ladies. In February 1817, the city council informed the managers that they viewed their efforts with pleasure and were disposed to aid them, pending a successful meeting. Accordingly, four managers promptly met the officials to provide such information as they desired. In May of that year, the city gave $500 to the women, who responded with a flattering note assuring the councilmen that "the approval of the wise is cherished with pe-culiar satisfaction." The state legislature also cooperated, first sending a dele-gation to inspect the asylum and then, in 1818, appropriating $2,000 for the home. Annual appropriations from the state ensued ($1,000 in 1819 and again in 1820; $3,000 for 1821), leading the women to praise "his excellency the Governor, to whom the Managers feel much indebted."[42] City and state in-creasingly depended on the women of Poydras for help in managing the con-sequences of poverty in New Orleans.

To the women's keen disappointment, the community at large consistently failed to match managers' goals for donations. After seven financially shaky years of operation, their institution continued to struggle, leading the secre-tary to scold in the annual report for 1824. "Useful, nay, necessary as such an institution must be in a city where Strangers, particularly poor Strangers have hardly found a location ere they find a grave, the Female Orphan Asylum has not received the generous contribution towards its support which might have been expected."[43]

In 1824, at the request of the city council, the managers agreed to accept two dozen girls sent by the mayor's office; Mayor Joseph Roffignac recipro-cated with much-needed funds, an annual stipend to the orphanage of $1,600. Although the reasons that led city officials to withdraw these twenty-four chil-dren from the Ursuline nuns' care and transfer them across Canal Street to the care of a mostly American Protestant board of managers are unclear, the city council had definitely heard rumors that girls at the convent were not properly cared for. Historian Emily Clark speculates that, in the new state of Louisi-ana, with its growing "American" presence, the primarily French-speaking city council may have repudiated Catholic caregivers to indicate "their fitness for American citizenship," thus demonstrating that they rejected fidelity to former French institutions.[44] On their part, the managers at Poydras agreed to instruct the newcomers in the principles of their respective religions, which necessi-tated hiring another governess to handle the Catholic catechism. Supportive of the asylum from the outset, the mayor had furnished enslaved laborers to cut ditches and maintain grounds at the home and had given other valuable as-sistance, prompting the secretary to record in her minutes that "the managers have great pleasure in being able to comply with any request of Mr. Raffignac [sic] from whom they have received many very important favors."[45]

Most lucrative of all, however, was the women's relationship with their early benefactor Julien Poydras, a tall and lean old man, slightly bent, with fine white hair and a grave, wistful expression in his dark eyes that seemed to hint at quiet suffering. For the last seven years of his life, Julien Poydras was pleased to spend many Sunday afternoons on the grounds of the refuge that bore his name. Dressed in the regalia of another day, knee breeches and silk stockings, silver buckles on his shoes and gold snuffbox in hand, he enjoyed sitting under the shade trees and watching the little girls at play. Sometimes he brought candy and toys for the orphans. Over the years, he gave steadily to the managers of the home, some $8,000 in all. In 1823, when he inquired about annual expenses, the society's treasurer, Phoebe Laidlaw, accompanied by two other managers, promptly sat down with him to offer detailed answers. They reported that, though Mr. Poydras was satisfied with their management, he regretted that he could do no more for the institution at present. However, he tantalized them with his parting remark that he "hoped before long to be able to assist it."[46]

Julien Poydras died on June 23, 1824, lying in a big, locally crafted cypress bed on his Pointe Coupée plantation, far from the New Orleans orphanage he had fostered. Such was the reverence in which the Female Orphan Society held the elderly bachelor that, immediately upon receiving news of his death, they directed that the orphans be put into mourning, ordering black armbands and bonnets trimmed in black ribbon to replace the usual uniform of domestic cotton pinafores and plain white bonnets. One month later, the board of managers received a copy of their patron's will and assembled in the asylum's parlor to hear the document read aloud. The women waited patiently through paragraphs detailing plans for the auction of the Poydras plantations, the provisions for future manumission of his enslaved workers, and his directions for the permanent care of his elderly slaves. One easily pictures the elation that surely gripped the dozen proper matrons when at last they heard the terms of Poydras's bequest to them. By his will, they were to be heirs to valuable New Orleans real estate, squares in the growing commercial heart of the American sector upriver from Canal Street. These lots on Tchoupitoulas and Poydras Streets, the three structures on them, and two more lots on the so-called batture, riverfront property at the foot of Poydras Street, carried a value of perhaps one hundred thousand dollars. In today's currency, the bequest would be worth more than three million dollars. If rightly handled, the rich inheritance left to the Female Orphan Society could allow the Poydras Asylum to expand and to thrive, serving generations yet unborn.

Beyond the initial generosity of its namesake, the Poydras Asylum benefited some fifteen years later from the largesse of two other major benefactors. When wealthy planter-merchant Stephen Henderson died in New Orleans, he left a generous but bizarre will, the arcane details of which need not concern us overly much. The will, probated in 1838, left explicit though highly convoluted instructions for the gradual emancipation of Henderson's slaves and for the creation of a new city on the upriver site of his Destrehan plantation. After some specific bequests, the document designated four New Orleans beneficiaries—Charity Hospital, the Firemen's Charitable Association, the Catholic Asylum for Destitute Boys, and the Poydras Asylum—to receive the bulk of Henderson's vast estate. Executors oversaw the partition of valuable commercial property (bounded by Robin, Front, Henderson, and Fulton Streets), which would yield a guaranteed income to each of the four legatees. The Henderson bequest included batture lands on Front Street below Henderson Street; these subsequently became hugely valuable, as the river was then 100 to 175 feet farther inland than it would be a century later. Some of these lands were later leased to the Texas & Pacific Railroad, and some to an entrepreneur who erected a mammoth and lucrative cotton press. However, tangled lawsuits over Henderson's will consumed time and a great part of his estate. A plentiful revenue stream did not immediately gush forth to assist Henderson's designated beneficiaries exactly as he had intended, but it managed to trickle and at times to flow freely, and the Poydras Asylum accordingly benefited through the years.

Another generous though unusual soul also remembered the orphans of New Orleans in his will. Alexander Milne, like Stephen Henderson a Scot by birth, had prospered greatly in business and real estate speculation in his adopted city. At the time of his death in 1838, Milne was the largest landowner in New Orleans, having bought up urban properties as well as twenty-two miles of undeveloped frontage along Lake Pontchartrain, stretching from west of the present Pontchartrain Boulevard eastward to the Rigolets. Though swampy, these lands yielding furs, lumber, and seafood were a basis of Milne's fortune. After providing amply for his two house servants and making bequests to relatives in Scotland, Milne's will directed that the remainder of his large estate, worth approximately one million dollars when he died, be divided into four equal parts. Two portions would go to found asylums for destitute boys and girls, to bear their benefactor's name, and two portions would go to extant institutions, one of which was the Poydras Asylum. Unfortunately, like Henderson's bequests, Milne's complicated will attracted lawsuits from disappointed kinsmen and execution of its terms was delayed for some time.

The bequest of Julien Poydras to the Female Orphan Society came seven years after the founding of the asylum; the bequests of Stephen Henderson and Alexander Milne came two decades later. Because of legal complexities delaying the transfer of assets, no immediate windfalls resulted from these three bequests; instead, protracted litigation ensued in each case because disgruntled relations challenged the wills of the three childless philanthropists. In time, however, the Poydras Asylum realized very significant inheritances from all three benefactors. The Poydras, Henderson, and Milne legacies went a long way toward relieving the asylum from the annual pressures of fundraising that, in the nineteenth century, plagued nearly all private charitable institutions for children. These welcome bequests meant that, with prudent management, the women of the board could ensure the future of the Poydras Asylum for the ages.

4

YEARS OF GROWTH

There was an old woman who lived in a shoe;
She had so many children she didn't know what to do.

Whenever she pondered the possibilities brought by the generous legacies of Poydras, Henderson, and Milne, each woman on the board of managers must have asked herself the same questions: *Will we have the wisdom to be good stewards of our inheritance? Will we manage our properties wisely?* Existing records show that, in overseeing the asylum's financial affairs, the early directors consistently displayed competence tempered with caution. It was not their way to make haste too quickly, but they were never timid. Though they routinely sought and received advice on legal and financial matters from husbands and fathers, all evidence indicates that they understood their affairs thoroughly; they alone made decisions.

In the year of their founding, dismayed to learn that the New York bank notes they had received as a contribution could be redeemed only at a severely discounted rate in New Orleans, they chose to ship the currency to New York aboard the brig *Fairy* in order to get a better rate. Learning from the treasurer's first report that annual receipts had exceeded expenses, they were quick to invest $1,000 in bank stock, and in subsequent years, they bought more.[1] When the financial panic of 1819 spurred many citizens to renege on their pledges, the group's income dropped accordingly. The secretary acknowledged hard times in her annual report, observing "the managers are well aware of the great pressure upon all classes of society in the last year."[2] Though not without sympathy, the women nevertheless hired a collector to pursue the promised funds. Practicality was a hallmark from the start.

In the early years, the managers undertook modest improvements to the house Mr. Poydras had given them. They fenced the lot, dug a well, enclosed a gallery for more living space, and fitted out another small structure as the widows' house; they added a smokehouse and a brick kitchen. However, as each year saw an increase in the number of girls requesting care, they soon faced an imperative to expand more robustly or begin turning away unfortunates. Their asylum had housed nine girls in its first year, but by the time of Poydras's death in 1824, it sheltered sixty-two children crowded into a most inadequate space.

Expansion seemed essential, but the law of Louisiana allowed the executors of the Julien Poydras estate to delay the transfer of property to legatees for as long as five years. While the managers knew they would eventually own real estate from which they could derive rental income, it was by no means certain when that revenue stream would begin to flow from their inheritance—not an ideal basis for making financial commitments. Nevertheless, the women met, less than a year after the death of Poydras, to consider bids for constructing a much-needed three-story building. At this time they undertook a full discussion of their assets and obligations. Although the necessity of having more space was clear, many managers harbored doubts and several expressed fears that their finances were inadequate. Then Phoebe Hunter spoke. While sharing their concerns and agreeing that strict economies would be necessary, she stoutly urged the group to go forward, reminding them that she "trusted in the continued blessing of Providence." Her appeal carried the day; the secretary recorded that, once she had spoken, "the managers hesitated not to make a choice." For the first time, and certainly not the last, the women of the Female Orphan Society borrowed money, empowered to do so by the act of incorporation. They obtained a loan of $1,100 from the Bank of New Orleans, and in less than a year, they had paid their builders in full. They proudly placed the document proving their payment in full among the "important papers."[3]

Thus, before the organization was a decade old, the Female Orphan Society's managers had exercised rights granted them by incorporation in order to borrow from commercial lenders. They had also employed attorneys: the women never shrank from litigation to gain their objectives. When the state legislature balked at appropriating more money for the asylum, arguing that the women should instead sue the Poydras executors to gain immediate possession of their handsome legacy, they instructed a lawyer to bring suit at once to hasten the property transfer. After negotiations, he informed the managers that Poydras's executors were ready to surrender the property two years sooner than required by law. Concurrently, the women themselves successfully pressed the legislature for help, insisting that "they really [were] in want of relief." However, when six weeks passed without the Female Orphan Society receiving a cent of the three thousand dollars that adjourning lawmakers had earmarked for them, four managers paid a call upon the governor to ask pointedly when they might expect to receive their money. A chastened Governor Henry Johnson returned the call a day later to assure them that the sale of gambling licenses would produce their money forthwith. On that occasion, the power of their personalities carried the day, and no lawyers were needed.[4]

Sometimes even distinguished legal counsel failed to gain favorable outcomes, as in the wryly humorous incident of the icehouse. The Poydras legacy included commercial buildings that the Female Orphan Society managers rented to New Orleans merchants. In the summer of 1829, B. W. Smith, who leased their Tchoupitoulas Street warehouse for use as an icehouse, wrote to demand remuneration for loss of his stock, which had melted while part of the roof was removed for repairs. The women were indignant. "Resolved unanimously," the secretary noted with feeling, "that the managers do not feel themselves justified in making any allowance or compensation whatever to Mr. Smith and feel much surprised that he should make any such application, the repairing of the house having commenced some months earlier than it would otherwise have been to oblige him, and with his full knowledge."[5] The injured Mr. Smith then served Phoebe Hunter with papers, announcing his intent to sue for damages.

Two local attorneys of considerable prominence volunteered their services to defend the managers against the suit, but, after hearing Smith's version of events, they advised the women to avoid trial by settling out of court. The attorneys were Thomas McCaleb and Samuel Livermore. McCaleb (1795–1832) was a South Carolina native and graduate of Princeton who represented the wealthy and eccentric John McDonogh in his legal affairs and served as counsel in every important case heard before the Louisiana Supreme Court for the seven years before his early death, in the 1832 cholera epidemic. Livermore (1786–1833), a New Hampshire native and Harvard graduate, was renowned for his extensive and valuable library on international law, which he bequeathed to his alma mater.

One wonders what Smith told the lawyers McCaleb and Livermore. The minutes make it plain that the managers believed they had acted on the merchant's own request in the matter of roof repair. The painful jolt of a $5,500 settlement was perhaps soothed somewhat by the fact that their attorneys had worked free of charge, but it constituted a steep financial obligation for a group whose funding remained precarious. In the aftermath, the women tartly instructed their counsel to inform the iceman that they would not be responsible for any damage to his ice in the future. When their lawyers produced only a mild document offering inadequate protection, the women unhesitatingly rejected it and instructed them to craft a stiffer agreement. When their legal counsel still did not deliver the stipulations they sought, the frustrated women prudently bought more insurance on the warehouse.

There was an unintended legacy of the icehouse fiasco: the disillusioned managers came to see their attorneys as fallible beings whose advice they need not necessarily accept. When Mr. Livermore, who had failed to shield them from liability for the combative Smith's melted ice, advised them to take a low offer for the rent of a lot of ground they owned, they thanked him politely but "after due reflection . . . declined to adopt his ideas." Instead, they hired an auctioneer and obtained a bid nearly double the lawyer's recommendation. In common with all women of their time, they had received a lifetime of cultural indoctrination in the fact of men's dominance and the deference they were owed, but this incident surely confirmed them in questioning assumptions of male superiority.[6]

There were other occasions on which the Female Orphan Society's managers found themselves at loggerheads with their lawyers. L. C. Duncan, a wealthy Yale graduate and prominent attorney who had ably represented them in several cases, actually tendered his resignation in 1839 because the women had the temerity to reject his recommendations; he huffed that they should employ a lawyer who would "command the undivided confidence of the Board." Duncan's letter prompted much discussion, with some members speaking vehemently about their right to dissent from any recommendation made by any individual, on any matter whatever. Fierce about preserving the ability to chart their own course, the managers nonetheless declined to accept

Duncan's resignation and passed resolutions reiterating their respect for his talents and integrity while also pointing out their "sacred right to approve or dissent." Their flattery having soothed his ego, Duncan agreed to continue as counsel. However, before the year was out, he had passed that duty to his brother Greer Duncan, who insisted on a resolution from the managers giving him *carte blanche* to act, in the Milne legacy suit, "either in court or out of court, and to take all such necessary and proper steps ... and to do whatever else may be thought requisite" in order to obtain the Milne bequest. The women agreed to his demand, "provided always that the same may be carried into effect amicably." This insistence on harmony proved too much for a member of the legal fraternity, and Duncan ultimately persuaded them to delete the limiting words.[7]

As the women of Poydras acquired more property to manage, they formulated a fixed policy regarding their holdings. In 1848, after more than a decade of complex lawsuits over contested wills, they rejected a purchase offer for a portion of their inheritance from Julien Poydras, property located on St. Charles Avenue and Julia Street. "The Management have always by a prudent economy endeavored to avoid *selling* their landed estate," the secretary noted. "They hope by doing so to lay such a solid foundation for the Poydras Asylum that it will always be able to extend its dimensions so as to meet the increasing orphanage of this growing city." This policy was not universally applied to their holdings, however. Though the asylum managers sentimentally held the Julien Poydras donation in reverence, calling it "the nucleus whence its [the asylum's] prosperity has steadily advanced," they willingly sold off lots left them by Milne, Henderson, and other benefactors if they deemed it financially advantageous.[8]

Once the property transfers finally occurred, the beneficent Poydras, Milne, and Henderson legacies allowed the managers "to act in an increased sphere of usefulness," as the secretary expressed it in her annual report for 1838.[9] Borrowing nearly $40,000 on the strength of their new holdings, they erected three more buildings at the corner of Poydras and Tchoupitoulas, which began to yield an annual rental income of $7,600. A few years later, they allowed two prospective tenants to build stores on their lots on Poydras Street and to occupy them rent-free, with the understanding that the managers would take possession of the buildings in five years' time. Eventually, in order to command higher rents, the novice real estate mavens built nine comfortable one-story cottages on their lots at the Milneburg lakefront. Because the village of Milneburg was then "out of town," they found it necessary to hire an individual to handle monthly rent collection there, paying him 10 percent of rents collected.

The real estate inherited from Poydras, Henderson, and Milne was chiefly undeveloped. This necessitated expenditures in order to erect commercial and residential buildings that could be rented for income, so that the managers regularly dealt with the need to spend in order to earn. In some years, expenditures were vexingly high while income was slight, a problem that continued to plague the board until their fortunes finally changed in the second half of the twentieth century. But, after a quarter century of a more or less precarious existence, the managers of the Poydras Asylum had at last settled into a reliable pattern by the 1840s, following a strategy of prudent but steady improvement of their rental properties and regularly going into debt to accomplish this. In this way, they created a revenue stream to finance asylum operations. Annual income was often uncertain; at times they failed to find suitable tenants for their properties, and at times unexpected expenses arose—for city-mandated paving costs, for example, or for newly imposed taxes. Nevertheless, the women's careful management of income and expenses ensured adequate financing and freed them from the unpleasant necessity of appealing for contributions. The secretary's annual report for 1851 offers a clear statement of the managers' operating philosophy and the strategy they pursued to achieve it. They held one object, "the establishment of a permanent income for the support of the Poydras Asylum. To attain this result great watchfulness in expenditure has been observed, real estate has been retained, and improved as fast as prudence will permit. When . . . the loans are paid off which the managers trust will be in a few years, this long desired result will be attained." Two years later, the report acknowledged "scrupulously counting the cost before every undertaking."[10]

By 1852, years of judicious management allowed the realization of the "darling hope of so many years," and the Poydras managers voted, confidently and unanimously, to construct an expansive new orphanage, "in a more retired situation for this family."[11] Their reasoning seems to have been based on a desire to go to a more nearly rural location, as the city was growing vigorously around them on St. Charles and Julia, bursting out of its original site in today's French Quarter and spreading into the American sector, or Faubourg St. Mary, as it was then denominated. The managers understood that their original location had increased tremendously in value and would be a lucrative source of revenue if rented to commercial interests. Divided over whether to build downriver or upriver from the city, the women visited potential sites. They rejected one in the rear of the city on the Pontchartrain Railroad as "pleasant but too remote," observing astutely that "an institution of this kind requires the protection of society."[12] Another, on the Carrollton Railroad some four miles from the city, they liked but deemed too costly. Other possible tracts were located out Elysian Fields Avenue, on Canal Street, and far out from the city on the Metairie Ridge. After enlisting a committee of four men to evaluate possible sites and make recommendations, they finally settled on a square of ground on Magazine Street, in a bucolic suburb then called Rickerville, some four miles upriver from the city, for which they paid $15,000.

In 1854, the women made their first payment of just over $4,000 on the chosen land. That fall, they treated the orphans to a dedicatory "Pic Nic" on the grounds, serving a variety of treats on tables in the shade and enjoying a pageant staged by the head teacher and her pupils. As children cheered, two "large girls" carried in the U.S. flag, a gift from their attorney Greer Duncan, and planted its staff, cut from a tree at Washington's Mount Vernon, in the soil. A self-possessed five-year-old dedicated the site as "the future home of the helpless orphan." The secretary's annual report that year summarized what the managers had accomplished at their original location. "Thousands of little unfortunates have been here sheltered from the chilling blasts of poverty—not only have their bodily comforts been cared for, but their tender hearts have been sheilded [sic] from the early acquaintance of vice to which their unprotected situation would lead them." Describing their new location as "extended, healthy, and accessible ... out of the crowded and distracting City," the report explained that the women had delayed in purchasing land, "being prevented from sooner undertaking it by prudence, their rule of action."[13]

The logical next step entailed selecting an architect. After considering plans submitted by three firms, they preferred the ideas of Lewis Reynolds, one of the city's most celebrated architects. Born in 1816 in New York State, he rose from the ranks of carpenter and by the early 1850s was obtaining his most impressive commissions in New Orleans. A peer of Henry Howard, Reynolds during a distinguished career designed large residences in Natchez, commercial buildings on New Orleans's Factors' Row, and at least ten of the grandest Garden District residences—notably, after the Civil War, the monumental Bradish Johnson House on Prytania Street, now the Louise McGehee School. The Reynolds design for the new asylum, estimated to cost $70,000, would produce a three-story building of most generous proportions, one hundred by two hundred feet, of Roman-Corinthian architecture. Initially pleased with their choice of Reynolds, the managers had reason to regret it before their dealings concluded.

Though the foundation was poured in 1855, the building would not be completed for more than two long years. Convinced that the old Poydras building they were vacating would find a lessee more easily if not occupied by over a hundred active young girls, the managers undertook the ordeal of moving the entire asylum to the Rickerville property in spring 1856, before the Reynolds building was complete. The children and staff occupied crowded temporary quarters in several old buildings on the grounds while construction of the new facility proceeded at a snail's pace. During this difficult time of transition, a pair of managers reported to the makeshift home every day to ensure smooth operations. Time and again, Mr. Reynolds vetoed their desire to take possession of the newly completed structure: first, the wet plastering stubbornly refused to dry, then, a leaking dormitory roof repeatedly needed repair. At last, after passing a difficult year and a half in cramped temporary housing, the girls and employees proudly occupied their new home in late 1857. Frugal as always, noting that they suffered "the same pecuniary embarrassment by which the commercial world is now so disastrously affected," the thrifty managers initially opted to forgo buying new furniture; instead, they had the old pieces cleaned and varnished. Shortly they relented, however, and ordered 150 iron bedsteads "from the North," plus new mattresses, at a price of sixty cents per mattress.[14]

A local reporter described the new facility in glowing terms, remarking upon its "neatness, massiveness, and beauty," which, in his view, had "no equal in the South."[15] Though life at the impressive new orphanage brought substantial advantages, such as improved bathing facilities, more spacious dormitories, and better organization for care and storage of wardrobes, it also delivered challenges. Because the location was so far away from the city proper, and thus from its engine companies, the managers cautioned the staff to be on guard against fire. The new situation required new rules. They forbade open lights and required all lamps and lanterns to be extinguished by nine o'clock, except in the nursery. They served the evening meal earlier, to allow time for clearing away the tables "before the necessity of candles."[16] Despite their sensible precautions, the threat of conflagration continued to haunt them because Mr. Reynolds had presided over installation of a defective furnace and inadequate flues. Three times the managers wrote to him to state the imminent danger of fire in the asylum; three times Reynolds ignored their letters. They obtained a report from the fire inspector who flatly pronounced the heating system unsafe. The unhappy reality of unheated dormitories and schoolrooms in January led the women to demand a meeting with Reynolds, who coolly failed to keep his appointments with them. Finally, in exasperation, they paid for rebuilding the furnace and hired workers to add adequate ducts for heated air. The records do not indicate whether they ever instigated a lawsuit against their seemingly deficient and definitely uncooperative architect.

Located well out of the city in what was then Jefferson Parish, the remote new asylum at the corner of Magazine and Peters Streets[17] was accessible in wet weather over unimproved streets so muddy that drays and mules coming from New Orleans literally became mired and immobile at times. In fact, when the new bedsteads arrived, the women chose to put them in storage "until the roads be in such condition as to allow of carting them to the asylum."[18] Sunday walks to church services were too far to be practicable, so the women arranged for a minister to come out on Sunday afternoons to deliver a spiritual message. On the other hand, the rural location and spacious acreage on higher ground near the levee allowed for cultivation of a large vegetable garden. The managers bought a horse and cart, kept chickens, and pastured cows at the property. Amply supplying their table with tastier and more nutritious fare, they soon had surplus vegetables and eggs to sell to their neighbors. Happiest of all changes for the children was the managers' decision to purchase games and install play equipment on the already shady grounds, which the practical women enhanced by planting pecan and orange trees. For years, they had worried over poor drainage on the muddy grounds at the original Julia Street location. The asylum's physician, Dr. J. Rhodes, had pronounced that low site "no fit and appropriate spot" for children and had urged the women to build a wooden platform above the bog as a dry and level place for play.[19] Not surprisingly, the 103 girls who moved into the new asylum delighted in their new surroundings. The grounds rang with shrieks, shouts, and songs as eager girls enjoyed every corner of the property, and the swings in the shade trees seldom hung empty.

Based on admittedly incomplete information contained in secretaries' annual reports, which in some years neglected to include a total in the key categories of admissions or withdrawals, it appears that the Poydras Asylum sheltered an average of 104 girls annually in the forty years of its existence at the original site, and a yearly average of 102 in the next forty years (1858–1899) at the new facility. However, there is a significant difference in the *total* number of girls admitted to the home at the original site and at the new location: a total of 1,342 admissions on Julia Street, contrasted with only 608 once the Female Orphan Society had removed to Magazine Street. The numbers of withdrawals likewise differ: a total of 716 girls withdrawn by family or friends at the original location, 573 withdrawn for the same reason from the Magazine house. Paradoxically, it would appear that the Poydras managers, with a larger facility, were sheltering no greater number of needy girls than they had assisted in their original home. Undeniably, they were admitting fewer girls than previously.

For explanation, we must acknowledge circumstances existing beyond their gates. For the first two decades of its existence, the Poydras Asylum had constituted the city's only orphanage for girls. The number of girls residing in the original asylum fluctuated from year to year. Then, in 1836, Roman Catholics opened their own facility for orphaned girls. (To the dismay of the Poydras managers, the new Catholic institution called itself the Female Orphan Asylum. The orphanage that Phoebe Hunter and her colleagues had created some twenty years earlier, in addition to being popularly known as the Poydras Asylum, was formally styled the Female Orphan Asylum. This duplication of nomenclature caused confusion at times.)

The work of the Sisters of Charity at the new orphanage relieved some pressure for admissions at Poydras just as great numbers of immigrants were streaming into the city. Beginning in the mid-1840s, each institution sheltered upwards of 140 children annually, a situation that continued at Poydras for the next thirty years. As the nineteenth century advanced, many other places of refuge for unprotected girls sprang into being, almost always affiliated with a religious denomination. By the late century, several other Catholic facilities were serving white orphans. In addition, there were the Protestant Orphans' Home, also called the Seventh Street Home, the Protestant Episcopal Church Home, the German Protestant Orphan Asylum, the Jewish Widows' and Orphans' Home, and several asylums that accepted boys only. For African Americans, the Thomy Lafon Orphans' Home housed orphaned boys of color and the Sisters of the Holy Family operated St. Mary's Academy, an orphanage for African American girls. In fact, New Orleans supported more orphan asylums than any other southern city. As capacity for sheltering orphaned girls multiplied, the demands on the Poydras Asylum eased. The total of residents in the new, more capacious Magazine Street facility in any given year reached a high of 157 in 1861, but as stated above, the new home operated with an *average* annual population of 102 for the remainder of the century.

As facilities to serve needy children multiplied, they frequently attracted the generosity of kind souls, but no one devoted herself to the welfare of orphans more tirelessly than Margaret Haughery (1813–1882), the celebrated "bread lady" of New Orleans. Confusion has grown up around the legend of Haughery, much of it concerning her association with the Poydras Asylum. Irish-born Margaret, orphaned at age nine when her parents died in Baltimore, never learned to read or write. Newly married in late 1835, she emigrated to New Orleans with her impoverished and sickly husband, but soon death claimed both her spouse and their infant daughter. Bereft and grieving in a strange city, she sought solace in her church and formed a special friendship with Sister Francis Regis Barrett, who superintended the Poydras Asylum briefly in 1836. (The story of the role of Catholic nuns at Poydras will be related fully in chapter 5.)

Some accounts hold that Margaret, who scrubbed as a chambermaid at the St. Charles Hotel to earn her living, also volunteered at the Poydras Asylum in return for room and board there. However, the meticulously kept minutes of the board of managers include no mention whatever of Haughery in the years when sisters staffed Poydras. A talented entrepreneur, she bought cows and sold milk in the city, steadily expanding her business and devoting the proceeds to aid orphans in local Catholic-run institutions. She purchased and

modernized a local bakery in 1859, making it quite profitable. Poydras minutes do indicate that Haughery sold loaves to the Poydras Asylum at four
cents a pound, a nominal price, allegedly explaining to the managers, "You are
working for the orphans; so am I. They are God's children, be they Catholic or
Protestant." Her philanthropy to children's asylums was legendary, and when
she died in 1882, her pallbearers included the governor of Louisiana and the
mayor of New Orleans. In a sign of respect, the Poydras girls were among
the many mourners who walked behind her cortege as it rolled through the
streets of New Orleans. Some sources, misled by the name Female Orphan
Asylum, have mistakenly asserted a long association between the generous
Margaret Haughery and the Poydras Asylum, but in fact, as a devout Irish
Catholic woman, she channeled most of her philanthropy through institutions
operated by her church. Her connection with the Poydras Asylum appears to
have been slight, on either of its campuses.[20]

The imposing new Poydras Asylum on Magazine Street gave more room,
indoors and out, to its young occupants, proved more healthful and satisfactory to all concerned than its predecessor, and drew approving comments
from the public. However, it also proved the source of an uncharacteristic
squabble among the managers that created deeply wounded feelings for a
time; as such, it provides a rare vignette of clashes within the usually harmonious board of managers.

To help defray construction costs for the new asylum, board president
Mary Luzenberg in 1858 appointed managers Margaret P. Adams and Eliza
Stringer to solicit financial contributions. The actions of this pair constituted
the first time since its founding that the Female Orphan Society had made a
broad appeal to the general population for contributions. Adams and Stringer
published a request for donations in the local press, alleging that the managers "need present and immediate help," urging that "if . . . each individual
gives his little or greater mite, according to his means, these improvements
can be completed." After a careful explanation of operating costs and numbers
served, the published plea closed pointedly: "Two thousand little girls, to say
nothing of poor widows, has this pioneer asylum rescued from poverty and
vice, and now fearlessly they lay their claim upon you, for *rescue* from their
present embarrassment. God forbid it should be in vain."[21]

The importunate plea shocked and embarrassed most board members.

Concerned that the appeal left an undignified as well as a false impression, the majority criticized Adams and Stringer vehemently. One particularly outraged manager asserted angrily that the unnecessary appeal made the well-endowed Poydras board a laughingstock, since it was commonly known that the managers owned valuable real estate in the city. Amid such scolding, Adams at last stalked out of a board meeting and subsequently submitted her resignation, though the board soon wrote her that they refused to accept it. Adams sent a letter of justification, reminding the managers that she and Stringer had been constituted a committee to raise funds and noting starchily that the public had a right to know the object of the aid thus asked. It was the placing of the appeal in public newspapers that triggered the heated reaction. Evidently when managers approved the appointment of Adams and Stringer to solicit funds, they had intended a discreet operation within the magic circle of friends and relatives. Asking the public for money when it was widely known that the Female Orphan Society held significant assets proved embarrassing to most of the managers.

Breaking an injured silence, Adams sent a second letter, expressing her gratitude at the vote of confidence from the board, which had declined to accept her resignation, and also avowing that she had heard that a Poydras manager had declared that "our needs were not what had been represented . . . at all." She wrote to warn the women of the dangers inherent in sending out contradictory messages regarding their institution's needs. And she wrote to demand, in cold dignity, an apology: "Still it is due to me, to my mortified wounded feelings . . . that the same lips that have done this great mischief should be the same to speak the words of correction."[22]

Who was the culprit who had so offended Adams? Evidence points to Phoebe Laidlaw. Shortly after the Adams imbroglio, it was Laidlaw who submitted *her* resignation, "respectfully and affectionately" but, most uncharacteristically for her, offering no explanation. She extended her hopes for the managers' future happiness and the success of the asylum and, after forty-five years of service, renounced not only her post as treasurer but also her position on the board of managers. The managers accepted the resignations, but to minimize the sting, they purchased a handsome and costly silver tray with two goblets for Laidlaw as a token of respect and appreciation. So trusted had Laidlaw been in the responsible post of treasurer that, as indicated by the society's minutes, board members had frequently voted her *carte blanche* in financial matters, empowering her to use her best judgment on rents and investments without consulting them further. But she was nearing seventy now and perhaps past her prime. Tellingly, the managers did not fight to keep her.

In choosing Laidlaw's nemesis Margaret Adams to replace her as treasurer, the managers selected strategically. When the long-serving Laidlaw departed, institutional memory departed with her; her resignation created a vacuum of knowledge about the financial dealings of the Female Orphan Society. The managers urgently needed expertise, and they gained it in the person of the new treasurer's husband. Thomas A. Adams, a prosperous Bostonian who had moved to New Orleans in 1842 and founded the city's mutual insurance industry, was then serving as president of the city's New England Society, which "surpassed virtually every other local club in the prestige and wealth of its membership," according to historian Frederick Starr.[23] The influential Adams almost immediately became the board's most trusted counselor on financial matters; managers sought his advice regarding nearly every issue that Laidlaw had handled herself. Adams gave his time most generously to the board, researching various questions and offering his sound counsel freely.

Ironically, the Laidlaw and Adams families lived within one block of each other on Prytania Street, a fact that must have contributed to the awkwardness of the situation after the blow-up. Adams, however, lasted but three years as treasurer before being ousted in a coup, flaming out with shrill written justifications of her several controversial actions, justifications producing more heat than light. She had chosen to defend some of her actions, at Laidlaw's expense, on the sacred pages of the bound volumes where Female Orphan Society minutes were carefully, and permanently, recorded. When members discovered that Adams had written uncharitably about Laidlaw's decisions as treasurer, their reaction was swift. They excised the harsh words and energetically defended their old colleague. Adams departed, and original treasurer Phoebe Laidlaw returned to her longtime realm of invoices and interest rates to serve for more than another decade.

January 1878 brought the first indisputable evidence of the elderly but still formidable Laidlaw's approaching death. Failing to submit her detailed annual treasurer's report on time, eighty-four and in poor health, she apologized profusely and promised to deliver it in February. On February 19, she called the group's secretary to her bedside and requested that she copy the carefully prepared report into the permanent minutes. The next day, Phoebe Hunter Laidlaw died, having devoted herself to Poydras Asylum business almost to the last hour of her life. Her death severed the last living link to the original board of managers. The Poydras girls attended her funeral, going first to her home to view her in her casket, hands folded and a peaceful expression on her faded face. Many wept openly; some leaned down and kissed her cheek. Comments that the girls later wrote in essays for their teacher reveal the fond esteem in which they held the veteran manager. "We will miss her coming into the schoolroom and we will miss her kisses also, and we will miss her telling us to be good girls and to be kind to each other," wrote Beatrice. Marie confided, "I hope that I will have another friend like her," while Pacquitta observed that the girls hoped to meet Laidlaw in heaven. She closed her remembrance simply: "I can write no more for I feel choked with tears."[24] Beyond doubt, Laidlaw was a regular and loved presence in the lives of the Poydras orphans.

With the exception of the brief interruption of Margaret Adams's controversial service, Phoebe Laidlaw had served as treasurer of the Female Orphan Society for an amazing sixty years. As a twenty-four-year-old wife and mother in 1818, she undertook to manage the initial $1,200 collected by subscription, and she continued as treasurer as, over the decades, her duties expanded exponentially. She it was who dealt with renters, lenders, and tax collectors; often, the board deferred entirely to her judgment about investments. Over time, the Female Orphan Society proceeded to serve hundreds of needy girls and widows; by prudent management, it remained solvent in spite of grave difficulties and successfully financed construction of a new asylum at a cost exceeding $70,000. In 1878, Laidlaw's Presbyterian minister noted candidly in his tribute that "her convictions and partialities were those of a strong and decided character," but he insisted that "they were exercised without giving offense." She wielded, he said, "an influence and authority which all who knew her were willing to admit and proud to uphold." In 1917, a Poydras board member struck a feminist note when she observed proudly, in her brief centennial history of the asylum, that Phoebe Hunter Laidlaw's sixty years as treasurer had concluded with "no man ever having written a line in her books."[25]

In their first century, the board of managers met, at a minimum, twice each month, and usually more often, at the institution itself. Because they clearly were loath to entrust any employee with true authority over the asylum's operations, no detail of asylum life was too minute to merit their attention. Not surprisingly, board meetings routinely consumed an entire day. The reminiscences of manager Georgia Mallard Seago (1865–1952) made that abundantly clear. She recalled that managers convened in the morning, paused for a simple meal at midday, and then resumed business. "Late in the afternoon they were served with milk and cake, after which they were driven home by their coachmen," she remembered, adding, "many a time the stars were out when our carriages started home."[26]

Notwithstanding a privileged status that included coaches and coachmen, the nineteenth-century managers were genuine workers with specific duties to dispatch. Some went regularly to merchants to make purchases for the home; others solicited competitive bids from butchers, bakers, repairmen, and gardeners; others executed a wide and necessary correspondence while still others prepared fact-filled reports for the board's consideration. Perhaps busiest of all were managers assigned to the visiting committee. They called at the asylum twice weekly during their two-month term of service, to investigate all aspects of the asylum's functioning. Beyond observing and inquiring, upstairs and down, indoors and out, they chatted with the children and the staff; they made their presence felt in a very real way by giving their time. Evidence indicates that, in the first hundred years, one manager or another spent some time at the asylum every day.[27]

The Poydras Asylum was a charitable endeavor of women, serving a special female constituency, but it required hard and unsentimental work. These nineteenth-century women managers wielded power, raising large sums of money and distributing them exactly as they saw fit. They were busy administrators: punctual, reliable, informed, and decisive. While caring for the needs of children through supervising a female staff at the asylum was not an unfamiliar role for women of the comfortable classes, they also dealt regularly with men of standing: architects, lawyers, bankers, merchants, and suppliers of all manner of goods and services. The Poydras managers were both tender-hearted philanthropists and hard-headed businesswomen.

When we consider the commitment that service on the board entailed, it becomes obvious that managers' daughters must have gained a keen awareness of their mothers' volunteer work for the Poydras Asylum. No doubt hearing their mothers tell of what they had observed and what they had done in their role as managers instilled in many young women a desire to emulate them. Throughout its history, the board of managers often turned to daughters to replace mothers; the minutes contain numerous examples of this passing of the torch of service from one generation to the next within a family.[28]

No example of continuity rivals that of the Hunter-Laidlaw family, however. Founder Phoebe Bryant Hunter served until her death in 1844. Daughter Phoebe Hunter Laidlaw's death in 1878 ended her sixty years of service, but a lineal connection remained in the person of Laidlaw's daughter Mary Ann (Mrs. William C.) Raymond. The board turned to the younger Mrs. Raymond to take up her mother's duties as treasurer. At her death in 1890, a fourth generation of the line of Phoebe Hunter, Hunter's great-granddaughter Phoebe Raymond Ferguson, assumed the treasurer's post and held it until her death in 1940 (although it appears that John B. Ferguson of Whitney Bank executed most of the treasurer's real duties for his wife during that time).When she died, the board selected her daughter, Mary Ferguson Greene, for the post. Finally, in 1941, after a century and a quarter of one family's female line serving continuously as treasurers for the Poydras Asylum, the line snapped when the young Mrs. Greene resigned her office, explaining that she felt unequal to its heavy demands.

This snapping of the string ended an impressive continuity, but fortunately the Poydras Asylum was in no way dependent upon any one family. Individual women would come and go, but the collective efforts of volunteer managers ensured that the home would endure. Indeed, it would prosper.

5

CROSSES TO BEAR

The Impact of Religious Strife on the Poydras Asylum

Now I lay me down to sleep, I pray the Lord my soul to keep,
If I should die before I wake, I pray the Lord my soul to take.

Each day at the Poydras Asylum began with prayer and scripture; each evening closed with the same. Poydras children learned to lisp their prayers while they were still toddling about in the institution's nursery. The vast majority of orphanages in the United States were denominationally affiliated and tended to accept children of one faith, either Protestant, Catholic, or Jewish, but for much of the nineteenth century, the Poydras Asylum went against the trend, admitting needy children regardless of their religion. Indeed, in some years Catholic girls outnumbered Protestants in the institution by a ratio of two to one. But the Poydras managers discovered that matters of faith could prove not only comforting and sustaining but also sharply divisive. The question of religion lay at the heart of one of the most painful experiences of the asylum's history, much to the regret of the earnest managers.

From the outset, religious instruction formed a significant part of every girl's experience at Poydras; the sincere religious devotion that underlay the managers' understanding of their mission ensured this. At the start of every board meeting, one of the managers offered a prayer, which was far from formulaic, followed by a thoughtfully composed devotional meditation enjoining her associates to greater and better service to God through addressing the needs of His children in the asylum. Only after looking to God did they address temporal matters of business. For the first few decades, Protestant and Catholic women served on the board of managers together, in an atmosphere of mutual respect and cooperation. When Protestants once unwittingly scheduled a board meeting for November 1 and then realized that it was "an esteemed and sacred day" for "many members of the Board," they canceled the session forthwith. November 1, All Saints Day, is a day of prayer and obligation for Catholics.[1]

At the asylum, the original routine for all girls included grace before each meal, twice-daily prayers with scripture readings, and Sunday worship at the nearby Presbyterian Church. This pattern shifted when the asylum welcomed twenty-four orphaned girls whose home had been the Ursuline convent. The nuns had long received a subsidy from the city for the care of indigent orphans, but in 1824 city officials abruptly determined to change that arrangement. Phoebe Hunter met with the mayor and city council members in October and heard the city's offer to pay the Poydras Asylum $1,400 annually for the girls' lodging, board, clothing, and education. Before accepting, however, the Poydras managers insisted on an additional annual payment of $200 to enable them to hire another governess. They intended that this employee would have responsibility for instructing the Catholic newcomers in their religion's duties and accompanying them to mass on Sundays, as well as serving as assistant in the schoolroom. Freely acknowledging having received from the outset "immediate and constant support from Catholic subscribers" to the Poydras Home, the managers felt an obligation to help children of Catholic parents to absorb the teachings of their particular faith.[2] City officials readily agreed to the extra outlay for an additional employee. Hasty preparations ensued, and five weeks later, the two dozen new girls settled in at the home, where the managers expected all to go well.

Almost immediately, however, dissension over religion became evident among employees and children, to such an extent that the managers found it necessary to formulate new regulations. Religious bickering had erupted among the girls, fueled by provocative comments from the paid staff. New rules soon mandated that employees must not "dispute about their different religions before the children or endeavor to instill religious prejudices into their minds."[3] The new rules barred night meetings and prayer meetings and stipulated that none but ordained clergy could come to the asylum to instruct children in religious duties, and only at the managers' request, hinting that perhaps priests or nuns or perhaps Protestant enthusiasts had begun proselytizing unbidden on the grounds of the asylum. They forbade girls to make visits off campus without written permission from a manager, this rule proba- bly indicating that newcomers were periodically finding their way back to the Ursulines' convent. Catholic managers and Protestant managers agreed on the necessity of restrictions aimed at ending religious rancor in the asylum.[4]

In thus restricting girls to the campus, the managers practiced an "isolating" model of institution management whereby they sought maximum social con- trol by shielding their charges from contact with outside influences. However, it does not necessarily follow that they were attempting to "save" girls from Catholicism, a charge often leveled at Protestant-operated asylums. Since they allowed girls of Catholic parents to learn the catechism, make a first commu- nion, and attend mass regularly, it seems more likely that all managers, recog- nizing that disharmony had flared when Catholic girls enrolled, blamed over- zealous Catholic clergy for encouraging the situation and, rightly or wrongly, sought to limit their private visits with the children while still allowing Cath- olic girls to practice the religion of their parents.

In the next five years, the managers experienced inordinate difficulty in regulating the asylum to their satisfaction. Frequent resignations of house- keepers and governesses contributed to a breakdown of discipline at the home, leading to what the minutes called "insubordination" among the girls. Much of the unwelcome turbulence stemmed from contentiousness over reli- gion. Indeed, the turmoil led the managers to resolve to admit no more chil- dren until smooth operations were restored. Meanwhile, they determined to hire a married couple to take charge, with the husband serving as a sort of headmaster in general charge of the institution and the wife as housekeeper. It seems clear that they hoped that the unprecedented step of introducing a man into the household would restore order. In this hope, they were disappointed.

After sifting through many applications and interviewing several couples, they hired a Mr. and Mrs. Edwards, but tranquility at the asylum continued to elude them. Mr. Edwards proved to be a prickly sort who clearly resented any glimmer of female will and found himself in constant clashes with women on the staff, frequently making appeals to the managers and complaining about employees' disrespect for his authority. Matters came to a head only four months after Edwards took up supervisory duties at Poydras. Wearied from his constant complaints against the staff, the managers held a careful inquiry to probe the accuracy of charges he leveled against Mrs. Sinnet, the sickroom nurse. They first allowed Edwards the privilege of extemporizing at length on her shortcomings. When he claimed that several staff members would validate his account, they then privately questioned each of them. While agreeing that Sinnet had a quick temper, they, to a woman, said nothing against her and maintained that she performed her duties toward sick children most attentively. The managers listened as Mrs. Sinnet gave her account of dealing with Edwards. At last, weighing what they had heard and discussing what they knew personally of Mrs. Sinnet from their regular visits to the asylum, they testily rejected Edwards' caviling and gave their nurse a ringing vote of confidence, labeling her "the most efficient person in the house." The emotional meeting was long and trying for the women, who concluded by addressing what they saw as the underlying problem. After much deliberation, they voted unanimously that they would not again give such authority to *a man*. The unpleasant episode had convinced them that "the experiment of having a gentleman at the head of the Poydras Asylum" had failed resoundingly and that such responsibility properly belonged only "in the hands of a respectable female."[5]

They had no qualms about hiring a well-qualified man as a mere classroom teacher, however, and in 1830 engaged Dr. John Kennicott, a twenty-six-year-old scholar from Buffalo, New York, who had recently come to New Orleans. Historian Thomas Conway labeled Kennicott "an opportunist with great hopes of getting rich or at least richer than one could expect to become in one's profession anywhere else."[6] Kennicott had landed the plum administrative position of director of all three newly created public schools in New Orleans, but evidently felt at liberty to enhance his income by contracting to teach a few hours a day at the Poydras Asylum. The feckless teacher soon disappointed the managers with his unreliability; after only a few months of classroom duties, he wrote to say that he would discontinue his attendance because his physician had recommended that he take a leave of absence during hot weather. The "medical leave" coincided with his return to Buffalo to marry his sweetheart that summer. Such a statement from the delicate Kennicott was the last straw for the peeved managers, who dismissed him and turned to a previously untried source for strength and competence in managing the asylum and teaching its children. They called in the nuns.

Early in 1830, two Sisters of Charity, an Irish-oriented order based in Emmitsburg, Maryland, had arrived in the city in response to a request from Bishop Joseph Rosati, who intended that they would teach free girls of color or help care for orphans. The Ursulines afforded them temporary housing in their convent, but evidently the newly arrived sisters found something uncongenial in either their living or working arrangements with the well-educated and notoriously elitist Ursulines. Tired and disappointed, they determined after a few months to go back to the motherhouse in Maryland. Providentially, just at that juncture, Poydras managers approached the Ursulines for assistance in operating their asylum. It seems to have occurred to the Ursulines' mother superior that dispatching the dissatisfied Sisters of Charity to take charge of the Poydras Asylum could be doubly beneficial, not only solving the Poydras managers' need for competent supervision at their institution but also giving the Sisters of Charity meaningful work to do, in a setting far across town from the Ursuline convent.

After Phoebe Hunter and four managers made judicious inquiries into the "habits, tempers, and acquirements" of the sisters, what they learned pleased them so well that they confidently urged the board to hire members of the order to take the asylum in hand. Frustrated by failure and nearly desperate for a smoothly functioning institution, the managers unanimously agreed to invite the sisters to Poydras, at an annual salary of $150 for each.[7] This move to staff the asylum with nuns must certainly give the lie to any assertion that, like most Protestant orphanages, the Poydras Asylum as of 1830 desired to minimize or weaken the profile of Catholics in the home.

Phoebe Hunter Laidlaw wrote the letter of invitation, which presumed that the nuns ("ladies who devote themselves to acts of charity and benevolence," as she called them) had already heard of the Female Orphan Society and its good work. Explaining that their capable staff was competent to dispatch the domestic side of running the home, but not its academic and moral aspects, Laidlaw stated that the managers wanted teachers "who would be impelled by a conscientious feeling to reside in the institution." Beyond classroom instruction in academic subjects, the job offer specified that the nuns would also care for the sick. To eradicate the reported outbursts of rudeness and ill temper that some girls had begun to display in the absence of a respected authority figure, the managers stipulated that the sisters would have general superintendence over the moral conduct of all. And, finally, they would of course attend to the religious instruction of the Catholic children in residence.[8]

Bishop Rosati's successor in New Orleans approved the request, as did the nuns' superiors in Maryland. Accordingly, shortly before Christmas of 1830, Sister Mary Magdalen and Sister Regina took up their duties at the home, which at that juncture sheltered twenty-eight children sent by order of the mayor and sixty-five admitted by other applications, making a total family of ninety-three girls. For the next six years, these nuns and others who came later shaped the day-to-day rhythms of the Poydras Asylum, bringing system, order, and enlightenment to the children and restoring serenity to a once-troubled institution. Yet, at the end of that time, their tenure came to a stormy close when they departed in high dudgeon, ending the Female Orphan Society's experiment with sectarian employees. The six-year episode at Poydras illustrates in miniature the larger Protestant-Catholic friction then afflicting the United States.[9]

In 1830, Catholics totaled not quite 4 percent of the entire national population; only thirty years later, the figure had ballooned to 37 percent. The great and rapid influx of Catholic immigrants into the United States from 1830 to 1860 constituted a rising tide of otherness viewed by many citizens as a threat to the fundamentally Protestant identity of the nation. Across the country, it brought forth unseemly backlashes based on ugly stereotypes and generalized fears. Samuel F. B. Morse, who would later gain fame as the inventor of the telegraph, famously wrote and spoke about his belief in a conspiracy by the Roman Catholic Church to eliminate the republican form of government in the United States, linking immigration and Catholicism, and making both seem threatening. The Reverend Lyman Beecher (father of Harriet, Henry Ward, and eleven other offspring) thundered his belief in Morse's Catholic conspiracy to all who would listen, arguing that Catholic schools were diabolical engines of subversion aimed less to educate than to win Protestant converts for Rome. In 1834, after the Calvinist Presbyterian Beecher preached three incendiary anti-Catholic sermons on a visit to Boston, firemen watched impassively as an enraged local mob burned to ashes the Ursuline convent in nearby Charlestown, Massachusetts. The convent had housed a fashionable school for girls, nearly all of whom were daughters of Boston's Unitarian elite. All of the men accused of the convent arson won acquittal, a decision met by courtroom spectators with boisterous applause.

Popular literature in the 1830s teemed with representations of scheming Catholic priests and nuns who committed shocking depredations against innocent girls under their charge. The "escaped nun's story" became a staple of fiction, describing the irresistible lure of Catholicism for unsuspecting Protestant girls. Drawn by the music, statuary, and rituals they encountered in convent schools, and often powerfully affected by the magnetic example of the sisters who taught them, some Protestant girls in these stories found themselves pulled toward the nunnery, the only path leading to full holiness and inner peace. But, their vows once taken, the innocents entered an unexpected life of horror and degradation, according to these publications. Susan Griffin, a literary scholar who has studied these once-popular books, recounts their general pattern:

> The protagonist is usually a young Protestant girl who has been lured into convent life. Often a priest (usually a Jesuit) has obtained power over the protagonist through the confessional, eliciting her secrets, invading her privacy, violating her innocence, perverting her emotions, and sapping her independence and will. Typical, too, are kidnappings in which the protagonist is bundled into a carriage in the dead of night and taken secretly to an unknown destination. Once in the convent, she is allowed no communication with her family, friends or lovers; all letters, for example, are intercepted or destroyed. Indeed, if those who love her manage to track the young woman down, the Mother Superior of the convent denies that she is present, sometimes claiming that she has died. Life in the convent is, at best, deadening and disillusioning; at worst, it combines sadistic "penances" with sexual violation (i.e. convents turn out to be "priests' brothels"). Daring clandestine escape offers the only hope for release.[10]

Among the most sensational anti-Catholic works published in this decade was *Six Months in a Convent,* whose author, Rebecca Theresa Reed, a young Protestant woman, had studied at the Ursulines' Charlestown school and intended to take holy vows. Soon disillusioned, she departed and, in 1835, published a gothic tale of the convent as prison, where depraved nuns meted out harsh and degrading punishments to vulnerable Protestant girls. The next year brought the vile *Awful Disclosures of Maria Monk,* whose young female author claimed to know, from experience, that predatory priests used secret tunnels to enter the convent, where they had routine sexual access to nuns.

The babies born of such liaisons were murdered, she revealed, but only after the sacrament of baptism. In fact, "Maria Monk" had never resided in a convent but had passed seven years in a home for wayward girls.

These sensational works enjoyed wide circulation; indeed, historian Richard Hofstadter asserted that Maria Monk's work was "probably the most widely read contemporary book in the United States before *Uncle Tom's Cabin*."[11] We do not know whether any Poydras manager, employee, or girl consumed so much as a paragraph, whether they heard others' accounts of the salacious writings, or whether they remained oblivious, but it is probable that there was some degree of awareness. The New Orleans press took negative notice of Maria Monk's scribbling, and the *Picayune* flatly denounced the book as "a tissue of false and malicious slanders from beginning to end."[12] Ray Billington, a leading student of nineteenth-century anti-Catholicism, sees a class basis for the consumption of such writings, arguing that middle-class, churchgoing Americans, like the Poydras managers, felt little attraction to the "violent sensationalism and frank pornography" of such publications.[13] Certainly, the influential Rev. Theodore Clapp, "the most independent minister of the Old South," in the view of historian Clement Eaton, frequently praised the energy and good works of local Catholicism from his Presbyterian pulpit, and many Poydras managers sat in Clapp's congregation.[14] The poison of anti-Catholic bigotry swirling around them seemingly failed to infect the managers; as will be seen, their actions argue against their having accepted this strain of prejudice. On the other hand, it is clear that Protestant staff members at the asylum, cooks, washers, housekeepers, and others, at times displayed a definite anti-Catholic point of view. Ironically, the Sisters of Charity, chosen in 1830 by Poydras managers to administer their cherished institution, were among the orders specifically mentioned in Maria Monk's hallucinatory horror. Yet the managers placed implicit trust in the sisters' judgment, and for the most part, the two groups of women interacted smoothly and respectfully during the six years of the nuns' supervision of the asylum (1830–1836).

Both the sisters' efficient management of the home and their unfailing ministrations to sick and frightened children during the severe cholera epidemic of 1832 won special praise from the Poydras board. The managers stoutly endorsed the sisters as "watchful and benevolent guardians" in the annual report for 1833, citing their "affectionate and attentive" demeanor to the children and the "flourishing state of the institution," which exhibited "in every department, order and cleanliness."[15] Attesting to their high regard for the nuns, they twice requested, successfully, that the Emmitsburg motherhouse send more sisters to help with "the family."

The sisters themselves spoke of their pleasure in working at Poydras, as letters from Sister Regina to Mother Augustine in Maryland testified in 1833. She asserted that the sisters were "as happy as the day is long in the midst of the sweet little orphans." She reported proudly that not only the managers but also doctors and visitors were "much pleased with the internal management of the house" and praised its "order, neatness, cleanliness." "Dear Mother," she asked, "if you had refused sisters to poor New Orleans, what would have become of these dear little orphans?"[16]

And yet, even as the home functioned properly, in terms of the girls' diet, cleanliness, health, education, and conduct, conflict between the nuns and Protestant employees smoldered and sometimes flared. The beleaguered managers held at least eight called meetings in five years specifically to address the contentious sectarianism at the home. Protestant employees criticized Catholicism and Catholics within the hearing of the girls, and the sisters returned the favor, each faction recruiting impressionable girls to their point of view. Friction between the sisters and Protestant staff members represented a longstanding motif, creating an ongoing situation that forced the Poydras managers to side with one faction or the other when they attempted to settle disputes. The minutes prove that the managers routinely dealt with the sisters with favoritism and for years gave almost automatic credence to the nuns' assertions in all disputes with non-Catholic employees.

Disputes between nuns and non-Catholic employees increased in 1834 with the hiring of Lydia Skinner, a teacher whose extra duties involved instructing the Protestant girls on religious duties. Only a few months into Skinner's tenure at Poydras, the managers were forced to call yet another special meeting to quiet sectarian bickering among the teachers. After inquiring into the situation, they recommended "forbearance and conciliatory measures to each party."[17]

Soon after this session, the managers confronted an odd problem. On the emergency advice of eight eminent doctors whom they consulted during the outbreak of a mysterious, unspecified illness among the girls, the board took

CROSSES TO BEAR ❧ 75

the extraordinary step of removing the entire Poydras population, at great expense and trouble, to live temporarily in another location. The physicians, four American, four French, had unanimously urged the move. Convinced by these experts that the Julia Street facility was unhealthy or contaminated in some way, the managers followed the doctors' advice and vacated the premises. The new temporary home, which they occupied for three difficult months in 1834, was seriously overcrowded and far from satisfactory, but at least there were no fatalities from the mystery illness. It was during this most trying time in makeshift, cramped quarters that the Sisters of Charity demanded a separate apartment for use as their chapel and accompanied the demand by a threat to withdraw their services from the asylum if it be not provided. The managers acceded, even though granting the request caused considerable inconvenience when space was at such a premium.

Once the difficult self-imposed exile ended with the return of the family to the disinfected asylum, the Protestant teacher Mrs. Skinner preferred serious charges against the nuns, alleging first that they "act[ed] in all things as though their principal object, and paramount duty was the conversion of the orphans to the Catholic faith." They accompanied their proselytizing with blatant efforts to instill in the children a sense of "dread and abhorrence" of Protestantism, she charged. Alleging several kinds of neglect and cruelty in her letter of protest, Skinner claimed that the sisters had confiscated and burned children's toys, forced ill-clad girls to scrub floors on cold days, and neglected the health and comfort of the orphans. Although the managers investigated, noting that Mrs. Skinner was previously considered truthful, the records do not indicate that they took her part, signifying that they could not verify Skinner's perhaps hyperbolic charges. Skinner was soon an ex-employee.[18]

Minutes reveal that, by 1836, the staff at Poydras consisted of seven nuns, "one man, three other [Protestant] females and a negress." Perhaps emboldened by their majority, the nuns now issued another ultimatum. Notified that the managers had found a well-qualified woman to serve as housekeeper and instructed to surrender the storeroom keys to her, Sister Magdalen flatly refused, threatening that all the sisters would leave the asylum if the new employee (presumably a Protestant) took possession of the keys. When called before the managers to discuss her reasons, the indignant nun indicated that possession of the keys represented the managers' confidence in her and that the call to give them up showed a lack of trust. In the discussion that followed after she left the room, some managers agreed that Sister Magdalen's feelings had been needlessly wounded and hoped to conciliate her. Others, notably the mother-daughter team of Phoebe Hunter and Phoebe Laidlaw, strongly disapproved of the sister's stand, with Laidlaw observing tartly that the nuns were assailing the right of the managers to manage the very institution that they had created. At length, the managers unanimously adopted a resolution stipulating that Sister Magdalen "is always expected with every other person employed in the Asylum to obey the directions of the Board . . . or withdraw from the institution."[19] In an effort to continue enjoying the nuns' competent service while asserting their own claim to ultimate authority, the managers had seemingly restored harmony at the home. In reality, the lull that followed was only an unstable truce. Unknown to the managers, a slow fuse was burning.

The disputed housekeeper Mrs. Clark came to work, on a one month's trial basis, and the sisters soon pronounced her an excellent cook and very industrious. Yet, puzzlingly, in less than two months, the managers dismissed Clark, citing "the want of harmony . . . in the institution owing to misunderstanding and disagreement between the sisters and the housekeeper," indicating again their propensity to defer to the sisters' wishes.[20] During or perhaps after this season of escalating turmoil, someone tore an entire page from the carefully maintained, leather-bound book in which Female Orphan Society minutes were recorded. This is one of only three instances of excision in the minutes' two centuries of existence, and hints intriguingly that something was recorded that, perhaps at a later date, cooler heads found regrettable.

Unfortunately, in the midst of this developing crisis, in May 1836, longtime board member Celeste Duplessis, a Creole Catholic, prepared to take ship for France, where she planned to remain for an extended visit of several months. Because custom dictated that board members tender formal resignations when they anticipated protracted absences from the city, Duplessis resigned. Her fond colleagues' resolution, passed to note her resignation, saluted "this assiduous and unwearied friend of the orphan" and warmly extended her "the united and affectionate wishes of her co-laborers for her safe return."[21] It seems possible that the absence of this respected Catholic manager during key debates diluted the patient spirit of ecumenical tolerance that had hitherto guided the board members as they attempted to quell sectarian rancor at the asylum.

In the summer of 1836, after the departure of Duplessis, Sister Magdalen notified the managers that she had been recalled to the motherhouse in Maryland and that her replacement Sister Regis would soon arrive. The managers met with Sister Regis to inform her that their resolutions were "considered important and [were] to be observed."[22] Noting the religious imbalance among the staff, they also announced to her their intention to reduce the number of nuns serving from seven to four in order to equalize the number of Catholic and Protestant employees. The newcomer countered with a letter insisting that seven sisters were essential to the administration of the asylum. Another and more significant part of Sister Regis's letter referred to the necessity of the sisters having a separate dining room and classrooms, citing "our rule which prohibits our having secular persons associated with us in our duty," excluding not only "Protestants but also Catholics and even our own relations" and alleging that the managers had long known of this requirement.

The minutes contain a lengthy reaction to these demands. The managers emphatically denied that they had known of the rules of the sisters' order, claiming that the nuns had heretofore only stipulated that they be allowed to hear mass daily. They noted a history of continual complaints, their long-standing tendency to take the nuns' side of an argument, and their pattern of routinely dismissing Protestant employees who proclaimed their innocence without having given them "that consideration which impartiality demanded." The tone of the minutes is starchy and sometimes irate.

The Managers feel every wish to do justice to what they believe to have been the kindness of the Sisters to the children, their attention to the religious duties of their charge, the neatness of the house. The *proof* of the estimation in which they [the nuns] have been held is their present assumption of power. They know that whenever the managers have directed any alteration in the domestic arrangements, they have only had to say the "Sisters will leave the Institution" and the change has not been persisted in....

It would not appear that the Board are to be *allowed* the privilege of appointing *one* person to assist in the duties of the Poydras Asylum, but she must submit to be excluded from the classroom and eating tables of the sisters, holding her situation as an *inferior,* which would of course lessen her influence with the children, and prevent her usefulness.[23]

On examination, it appears that the managers failed to understand or honor Catholic regulations governing the nuns' daily routine. It also appears that the sisters had not insisted on strict observance of all regulations since their arrival in 1830. However, the managers were being less than forthright about what they had understood about those rules. In 1832, after two serene years at Poydras, Sister Regina had informed the managers that her superiors had made known to her that "implicit observance of their rules is now required." The managers then wrote to Emmitsburg, requesting special dispensation for their Catholic employees to continue to work in close conjunction with Protestants. They expressed themselves highly appreciative of the sisters' service, reminded the officials that their institution served both Catholic and Protestant girls, and noted pointedly that their board at that time consisted of equal numbers of Catholic and Protestant managers. Evidently they received the exemption they sought. Solid evidence for this interpretation exists in an 1847 letter to Bishop Antoine Blanc, in which one Sister Lorretta, looking back on her time at the Poydras Asylum, confided to him that "if she had not been under vow she would not have remained," because "there was anything but rule kept."[24] Thus, the managers' reaction of surprise on learning that the nuns' mingling with Protestant staff at mealtime violated a rule of their order does not ring true, since only four years prior, they had addressed the same issue when they wrote to appeal for an exception.

The nuns serving at Poydras were Sisters of Charity. Women in this order, founded by Mrs. Elizabeth Bayley Seton in Emmitsburg, Maryland, in 1809, did not wear the veil, nor were they cloistered. Instead, their dress featured a simple black cap with a black cape, similar to a widow's garb. Vincent de Paul, who founded the Daughters of Charity in Paris in the seventeenth century, had originally intended the women to work in the community among the sick and poor. Because he knew that they would find life in the cloister incompatible with their mission, he decreed that they would have "no cloister but the streets of the city or the wards of the hospital, no enclosure but obedience, no grate but the fear of God, no veil but holy modesty." Catholic superiors had permitted exceptions to an order's rule on many occasions; indeed, obtaining permission to deviate was not at all unusual in the challenging conditions of the nineteenth-century United States. For example, in Louisiana, nuns had won permission to use English rather than Latin for children's prayers. Sisters seem to have sought dispensations when the rules were serious hindrances to their mission, but there was no clear stance among nuns on this issue; some felt strict observance of every detail was essential, while others believed some changes were for the best. The final decision always rested with the sisters' superiors. During the Civil War, Frederick Law Olmsted reported having seen forty nuns on a hospital boat who refused to lift a hand to help the sick and wounded; a priest had forbidden them to do so because, in violation of the rule, there was no chapel set up for their use. When the priest, their ecclesiastical superior, objected, the nuns, who had taken a vow of obedience, obeyed. We do not know how they felt about the situation. Nor can we know, at this remove, how the nuns at Poydras felt about sharing a small dining room at mealtime with Protestants; we cannot know whether they preferred to have that portion of their rule suspended so that they could continue to work among the Poydras orphans or whether they preferred strict observance.

The surprising denouement of the ceaselessly simmering squabble at Poydras came in October 1836. Giving a mere two weeks' notice to the managers, the nuns, on orders from their superior, shocked the board by announcing their complete and permanent withdrawal from Poydras Asylum. A perfect storm of difficulties then converged, as the institution's cook gave her notice and announced she would leave with the sisters. Evidently feeling the need to begin afresh, the managers cleared the deck fully by discharging other employees, leaving them with over one hundred children and the necessity of procuring an entire staff of matron, nurse, teachers, cook, and washer—a task they completed with only two days to spare. When the managers requested, for their records, a copy of the letter Sister Regis had read them, demanding separate facilities for the nuns, she refused, stating that her superior, the Rev. Augustine Jeanjean, would not allow it, surely an indication of ill will.

At this remove, it is difficult to know what exactly occasioned the withdrawal of the nuns from Poydras. As millions of Irish immigrants arrived in the overwhelmingly Protestant United States, Irish Catholic clergy in the United States displayed a strong and well-documented preference for "saving" Catholic children from the presumably pernicious influence of Protestant organizations. Catholic fears of Protestant proselytizing were strong and long-lasting—and, in many cases, well-founded. Msgr. John O'Grady, longtime executive secretary of the National Conference of Catholic Charities, asserted in 1930, "When the friendless children of the Irish were brought to them [Protestants], their only thought was to preserve them from the errors of 'Romanism.'"[25] The Roman Catholic hierarchy in New Orleans had begun operating St. Mary's, an asylum for orphaned boys, in 1835. Irish-born priest Adam Kindelon headed the boys' orphanage. He confided to his bishop in the summer of 1836, a few months before the nuns' departure from Poydras, that things were going well for the Catholic church in New Orleans, "with the exception of the Poydras Asylum, the lady managers as usual giving trouble to the poore [sic] sisters."[26] A belief, held against considerable evidence to the contrary, that children at the Poydras Asylum were in danger of being lost to the Catholic faith, certainly contributed to the Catholic leaders' decision to establish their institution for girls in "The Withers," an old house on New Levee Street (today South Peters Street). Smoldering animosity may have been equally animating. Perhaps motivated by spite over the pattern of clashes between nuns and Protestant staff at Poydras, church leaders and the sisters coolly gave only the most minimal advance notice of their plans to the Poydras managers.

Exactly two weeks after the nuns' bombshell burst, the Poydras children assembled in the schoolroom for roll call. Phoebe Laidlaw addressed them, stressing the necessity for gratitude to the sisters for their kindness and attention and entreating them to behave properly during the time of transition. The children, some 119 in all, promised obedience, no doubt encouraged by Laidlaw's promise of rewards for good conduct at Christmas. Sister Regis then went over the house with the new employees and the managers, "politely affording every information in her power," and then the sisters quietly took their leave of Poydras Asylum.[27] It appeared that all had been done that should be done, leading the managers to expect a serene transition.

Ten days after the nuns' departure, however, the managers found it necessary to meet in special session to address a situation of outright rebellion in the asylum. Unknown to them, in direct violation of the asylum's protocols, the Catholic girls at Poydras had, for quite some time, refused to remain in the schoolroom when portions of the New Testament were being read, having been forbidden to listen by the fiery Father James Ignatius Mullen, they said.

On the first Sunday evening of the new employees' tenure, Catholic girls had entered the schoolroom along with Protestants when the bell was rung for devotionals, as per routine, but the minutes record that suddenly "they [Catholics] all rose with great noise and confusion and rushed from the room exclaiming 'Protestant Bible'... and ... they continued running up and down stairs in great disorder and tumult[;] several hours elapsed before, in any degree, order could be restored."[28]

In the wake of the mini-riot at the asylum, Catholic members of the board of managers explained to their Protestant colleagues that, in their view, there was misunderstanding on the part of the girls about what Father Mullen had said regarding allegedly prohibited scriptures. While the Catholics' Old Testament differed from that used by Protestants (it contained more books, including the so-called Apocrypha), Catholic managers maintained that the New Testament was never prohibited in Catholic services; indeed, they were at pains to note that it was used "by their church and in their families."[29] However, unlike the latitudinarian Catholics on the Poydras board, some Catholics of stricter persuasion held that, due to allegedly false translation, the King James Version of the Bible wrongly omitted certain passages and included others that did not belong in scripture. Such Catholics viewed only the sixteenth-century Douay-Rheims translation from the Latin Vulgate as acceptable. Whether instructed by the sisters or, more likely, by their recently arrived Irish priest, the militant Father Mullen of St. Patrick's Church, the Catholic girls at the asylum in the mid-1830s had clearly imbibed a belief that the "Protestant Bible" was not in accord with devout Catholicism. This represented a sharp departure from the previously harmonious approach to scripture readings, wherein for years all girls, Catholics and Protestants alike, had participated.

The managers summoned the girls, gravely reprimanded them for their boisterous display, and enjoined them to obey the rules of the asylum. However, they soon learned, to their dismay, that, to avoid conflict with an outspoken contingent of intransigent older Catholic girls, the staff, in the managers' absence, chose not to force them to listen to the "Protestant Bible" and instead abandoned the longstanding practice of requiring all to attend twice-daily scripture readings.

Meanwhile, more religious conflict flared when a Poydras child about ten years old secretly left the asylum and made her way, during a hard rain, to the newly established Catholic female orphanage, staffed by the sisters. This child, Mary Handloft, had been registered as Protestant when she entered with her two sisters, but during a severe illness, of which one of her sisters had died, she was baptized by a priest at the request of the nuns attending her. When she recovered, she had regularly attended Catholic services. The managers reported themselves shocked at her disobedience in leaving her home with them and also were "much aggrieved" when the nuns refused their written request to return Mary to Poydras. A delegation of Poydras managers called at the Catholic orphanage to claim Mary, but the nuns responded that the child wished to stay with them and that they would not willingly release her. They added slyly that "the ladies had their permission to enter their house and take the child by force if agreeable to them," which offer the managers promptly declined. Nevertheless, they persisted for three full months, unsuccessfully, in their efforts to reclaim Mary and reunite her with her only surviving sister, a Protestant who lived at Poydras.[30]

In order not to alarm subscribers and potential donors, the secretary's annual report for 1836 intentionally minimized the year of religious strife that had shaken the managers and their institution. The document falsely asserted that "happiness and harmony reign[ed]" at the home. Though written only a month after the clash over the young runaway, two months after the "Protestant Bible" riot, and three months after the nuns had forsaken the asylum, the summary omitted all mention of Protestant-Catholic turmoil, noting only that the nuns had left because of the rules of their order.[31]

In the years before the Civil War, far from attempting to produce religious orthodoxy or adherence to Protestantism among the girls, the managers seem to have made strenuous efforts to rear the children in the respective faiths of their parents, if known. Each year, they paid to have white dresses made for Catholic girls who made a first communion. They arranged for staff to accompany the children to Protestant or Catholic worship services on Sundays. They assigned a teacher to instruct the girls in the duties and doctrines of their respective religions, and they set aside money to purchase appropriate religious books for each set. Yet the conflict over religion simmered on, boiling over again on the issue of placing girls in families whose religion they did not share. The board of managers had attempted to place Catholic girls with Catholic families, and Protestant with Protestant, but this was not always possible. When good family situations presented themselves, they ignored religious preference and placed girls, motivated by their belief that a genuine home with a responsible family carried more importance than honoring religious preferences of deceased or absent parents.

As the years passed, the Poydras managers increasingly resented Father Mullen, the confrontational Irish-born priest who offended them by his interference and criticism of their placements. Described as "big, forcible, outspoken [and] rough," he had fired off a hot letter in which he fulminated against them as a "Board of Protestants," demanded that a child be removed from a Protestant family and a Catholic family found for her, and threatened "they shall hear something from me on the subject that will not be very agreeable to them." Mullen further accused the managers of "kidnapping," thundering "we shall not tamely submit to such bigoted proselytion [sic] by Protestants."[32] The managers fumed over the priest's tendency to try "to dictate to this Board" and, in response, passed a tart resolution in February 1848, less than a month after receipt of Mullen's complaint, in which one hears the managers' growing irritation over the religious question.

Resolved, that whereas many worthy persons who take these friendless orphans with the conscientious intention of acting kindly and faithfully toward them, are occasionally so annoyed on the subject of the religion of the children, by their friends and relatives (who are neither able or willing to take care of them) as to be compelled either to return them to the Asylum or to appeal to the Managers for redress. It is therefore the opinion of this Board that the Managers (not being bigoted) are fully qualified and authorized to make such disposition of the children placed in the institution, as their judgment may direct to place them with any family who may be considered by the Board qualified to rear them as moral and useful members of society, without any regard to the particular religious denomination to which such family may belong. And that this resolution be fully understood by all who desire to place their children in this institution before they be recieved [sic] into the house, and that for the *present*, each child shall attend the church in which she was baptized, but it shall rest alone upon the judgment of the Managers where she shall subsequently be placed, whether with Protestant or Catholic, as they may decide.[33]

The next decade of the 1850s witnessed a vigorous flowering of nativism in New Orleans. The dire famine that gripped Ireland from 1845 through the mid-1850s caused perhaps one million men, women, and children, nearly all of whom were Catholics, to flee, literally for their lives. As one of the chief entry ports for European immigrants to the United States, New Orleans faced a situation without parallel in the rest of the South. The white foreign-born population of Louisiana in the mid-1850s, most of whom resided in the Crescent City, numbered over 26 percent of the state total, while, by contrast, neighboring Mississippi counted only 1.61 percent foreign-born residents. Indeed, in the 1850s, only New York received more immigrants than New Orleans. This population equation helped to fuel a robust nativism among New Orleanians. The American or "Know-Nothing" Party, a national movement characterized by anti-Catholic, anti-immigrant sentiments, gained considerable strength in the city in this decade. During 1854, New Orleans streets rocked with vicious riots between Irish immigrants and Know-Nothings, and in that year, Know-Nothing candidates swept to power in the city's municipal elections.[34]

True, New Orleans had boasted a very large Catholic population prior to the Irish influx, but the great majority of these native Catholics were Louisiana-born Creoles. Creole Catholics on the whole took a markedly more moderate, relaxed approach to their religion and mistrusted the ultramontane and less flexible Catholicism of the Irish. The latter quite vocally favored the assumption of political and secular authority by the pope, a position at odds with the Creoles' opposition to what they saw as papal overreach. Historian Randall Miller notes that Irish and Creole Catholics "did not always honor the same religious heroes or stress the same private devotions. They did not preach, or want preached, the same kind of sermons."[35] Judging by given names and surnames, there were Catholic Creoles on the Poydras board of managers, inclined neither to proselytize nor to distrust Protestants, a fact that no doubt fostered harmony between Protestant and Catholic members of the board in the antebellum years.

Yet the Poydras Asylum in the 1850s proved to be a sectarian combat zone where Catholic-Protestant tensions flared just as they did in New Orleans at large. Once again, employees at the home contributed manifestly to the frictions, Catholic workers showing contempt for Protestantism and Protestant workers the same contempt for Catholicism, with many staffers recruiting girls as clients for their particular prejudices. So inflamed had the situation become that some Catholic girls refused to join in "with the family in offering daily thanks to their Creator," obviously having been persuaded that Catholics and Protestants should not pray together. Some now displayed what the secretary called "the sad delinquency" and "spirit of insubordination" that led them to refuse even to repeat the Lord's Prayer as well as to avoid morning service where a teacher read passages of scripture.[36] When runaways continued to visit the convent and returned more recalcitrant than ever, the managers expressed a belief that nuns had induced them to absent themselves. They concluded that their former policy of allowing unsupervised "large girls" to go out from the asylum on errands must now end.

For some years, the women of the Poydras board, most of whom were wives and mothers, worked successfully with nuns in the operation of their institution, finding much to admire in the sisters' competent management. No doubt the Protestant board members had found the nuns' practices of celibacy and communal living somewhat odd, when their own society insistently prescribed marriage, motherhood, and domesticity for every woman. Quite likely they sometimes looked askance at the nonconformity of these independent women, who, by choosing not to marry, bear children, or establish homes of their own, subverted gender norms and presented a different model of adult womanhood. Yet the Poydras managers were, for their own society, presenting another quite different model of adult womanhood, in their frankly independent management of real estate and handling of money. Perhaps their own unusual degree of autonomy made it easier for them to work with the sisters. Certainly, for the sake of system and order at the asylum, the board members had overcome any hesitations they might have had about close cooperation with such unconventional women, and consequently, the cooperation between nuns and managers at Poydras had, for a time, defied the stark denominational pattern that prevailed at nearly all nineteenth-century American orphanages.

However, scarred by bitter experience, the managers eventually came to believe that a proselytizing Catholic influence spawned disharmony in the asylum and was harmful to their mission. Mourning the absence of kindliness and tolerance among the asylum's staff and girls, the managers gravely admitted that they "kn[e]w not how to reconcile or exclude the spirit of antagonism."[37] To their great dismay, the Catholic-Protestant enmity then roiling the country at large had taken root under their roof.

As a last resort, the historically tolerant Poydras board of managers, whose city had a long tradition of interfaith acceptance, held a lengthy discussion of the propriety of employing Catholic staff in the home. After over four decades of hiring with little regard to religion, they voted, in a decision not taken lightly, that in the future they would make every attempt to hire none but Protestants. Rightly or wrongly, they blamed their adult working-class Catholic employees for igniting and stoking religious disputes among the girls, and they blamed nearby Catholic clergy for encouraging the discord. The managers left the admissions policy unchanged, however, and the Poydras Asylum continued to admit girls of all faiths. Indeed, in many years, Catholic girls would outnumber Protestants in the home. The received wisdom that Protestant institutions energetically strove to convert Catholic children does not readily apply to the Poydras Asylum.

Were the managers motivated by religious prejudice? It is surely possible, though convincing evidence is lacking. But it is certain that sheer weariness with the ongoing, seemingly chronic religious dissension among disputing staff members, which spilled over and infected impressionable girls, brought the exasperated board to adopt their draconian policy. They wanted a restoration of peace.[38]

And the new regulation did bring peace to Poydras, but beyond the gate, peace was breathing its last.

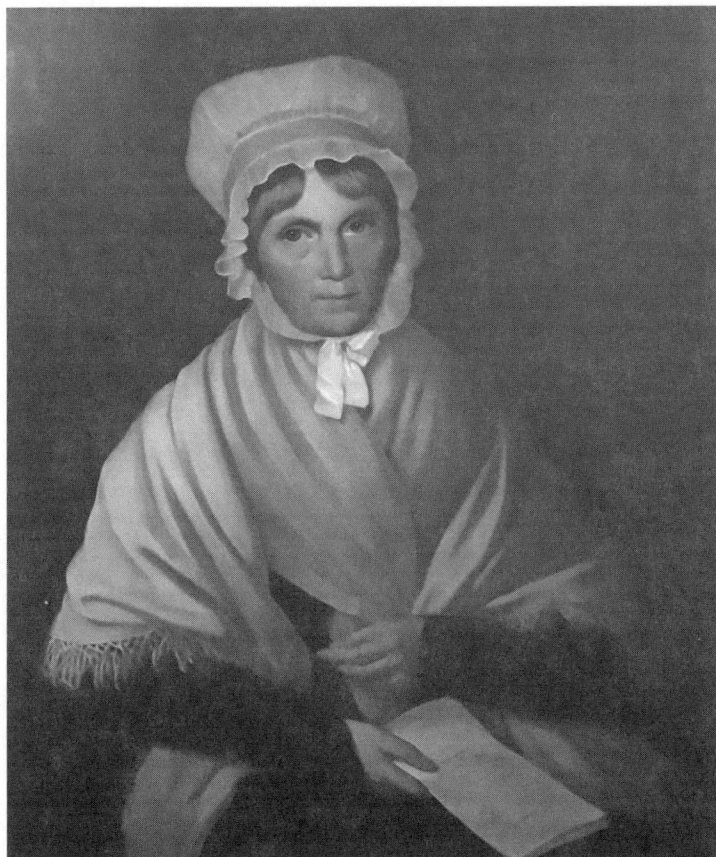

Posthumous portrait of Phoebe Bryant Hunter, founder of the Female Orphan
Asylum in New Orleans, painted by Francisco Bernard.

Poydras Home Archives

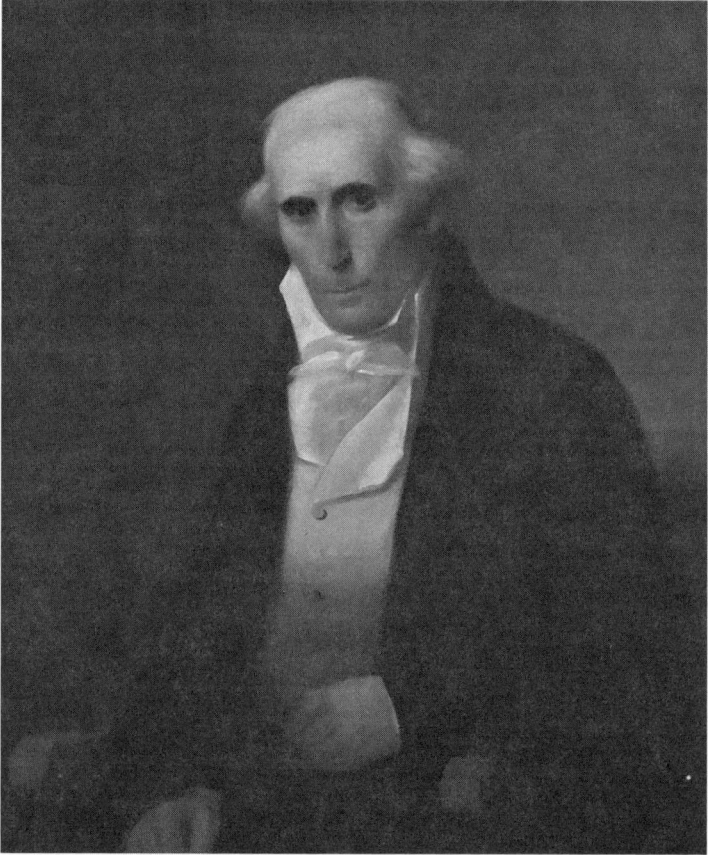

Portrait of Julien Poydras, attributed to William Edward West, 1820.
Poydras Home Archives

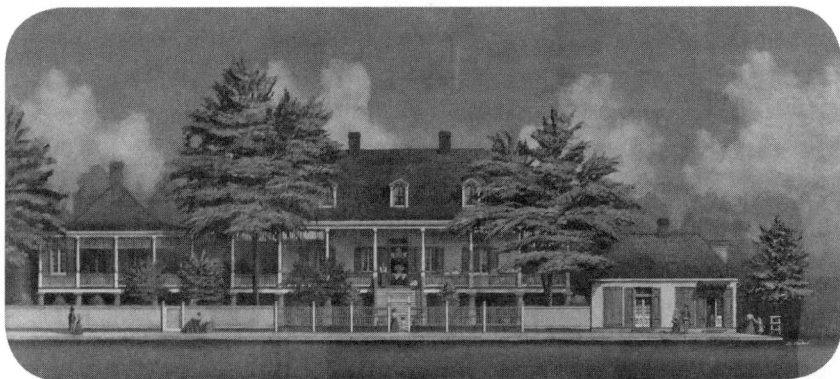

The New Orleans plantation home of Julien Poydras,
which he donated to the Female Orphan Society. It served as the first Female
Orphan Asylum, also known as the Poydras Asylum, 1817–1857.
Poydras Home Archives

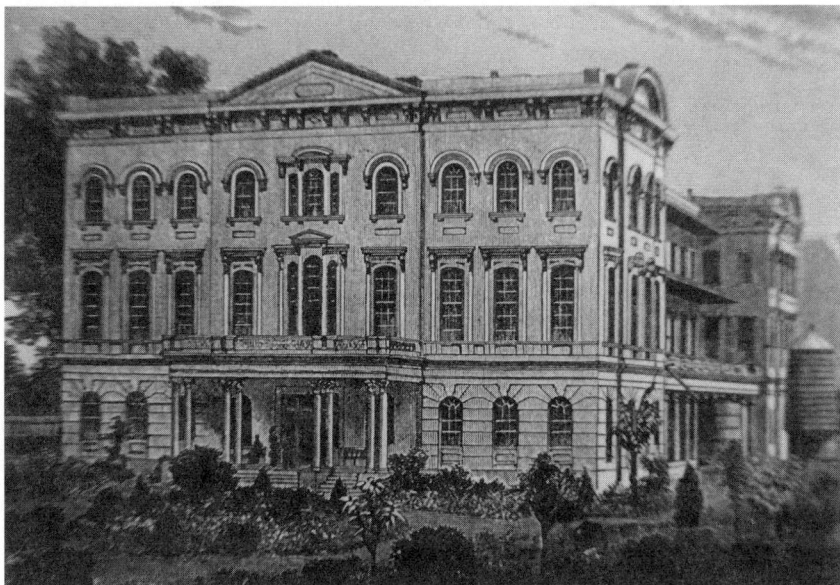

Architectural drawing of the second Poydras Asylum, built in 1857.
Poydras Home Archives

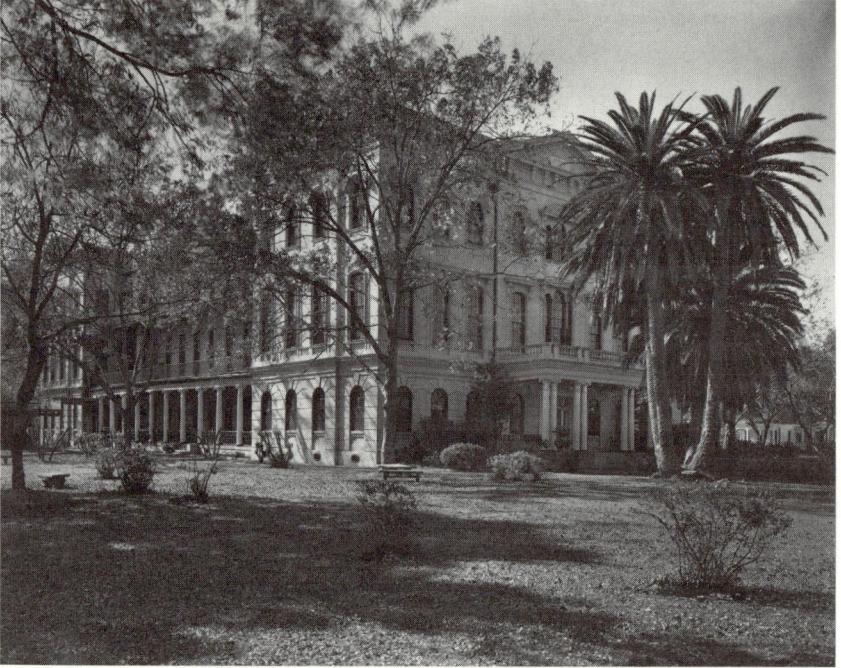

The second Poydras Asylum, located at Magazine and Peters
(now Jefferson Avenue). Designed by renowned architect
Lewis Reynolds; completed 1857.
Poydras Home Records, Louisiana Research Collection, Tulane University

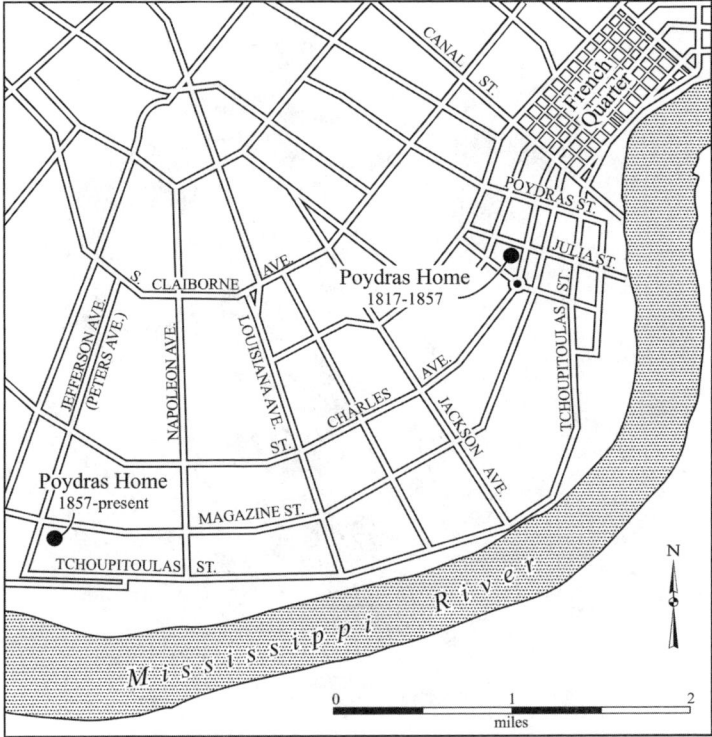

Original and present locations of the Poydras Asylum.

Map by Mary Lee Eggart

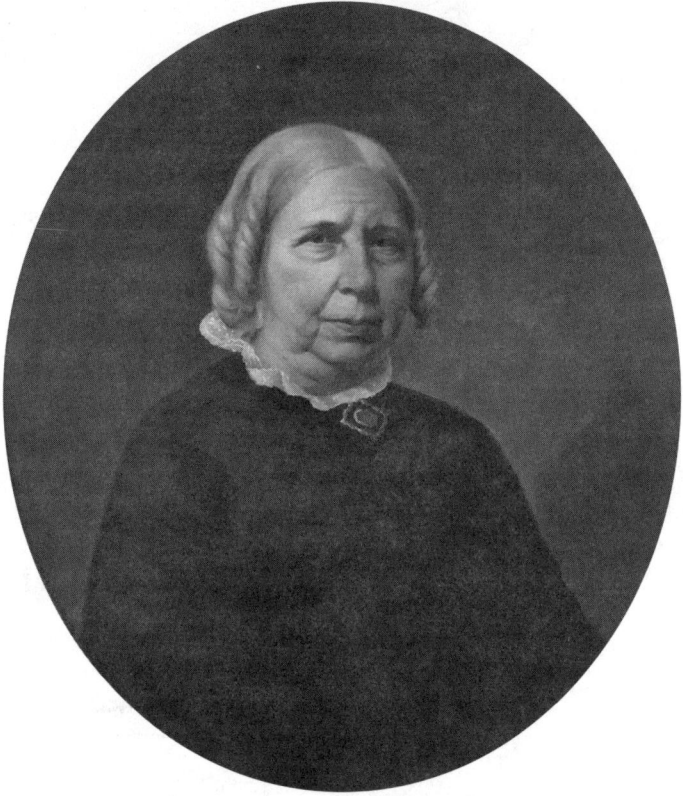

Clemence Toby, board member and directress of the Poydras Asylum, 1838–1879.
Poydras Home Archives

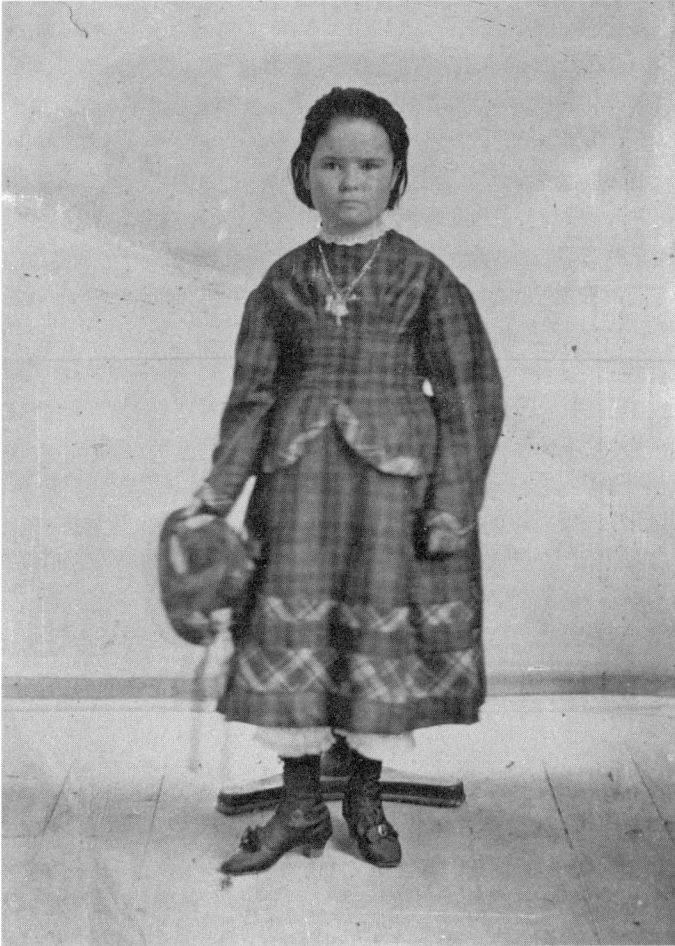

Unidentified girl who resided at the Poydras Asylum.
Poydras Home Records, Louisiana Research Collection, Tulane University

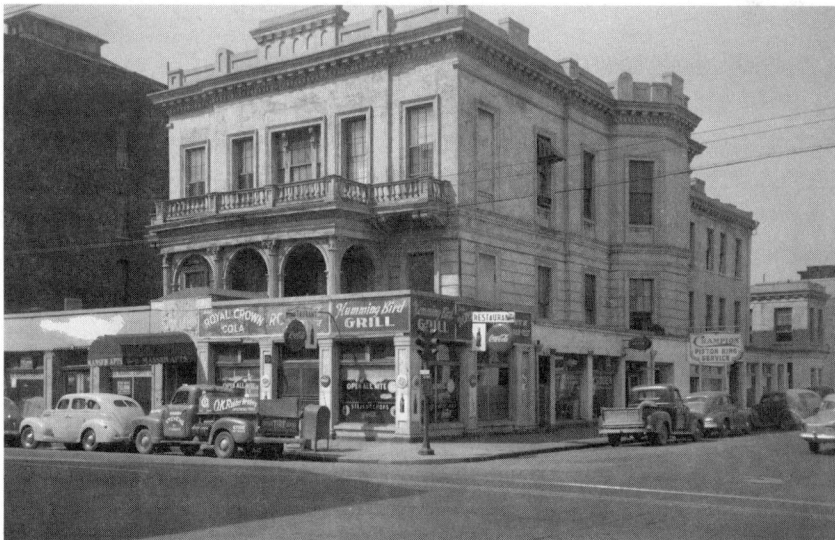

The home of Dr. George Campbell, built in 1859 at St. Charles and Julia Streets, on land leased from the Poydras board of managers. By the time of this mid-twentieth-century photograph, the board was operating the once-elegant structure as the Mansion Apartments.

Louisiana Division/City Archives, New Orleans Public Library

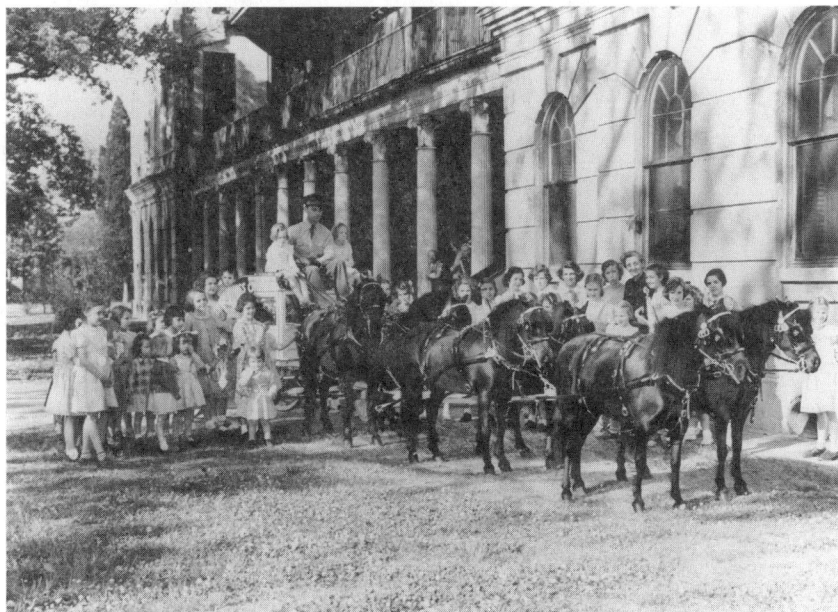

A local dairy's miniature milk wagon, pulled by ponies, with some of
the Poydras children in front of the Poydras Asylum, c. 1940.
Poydras Home Archives

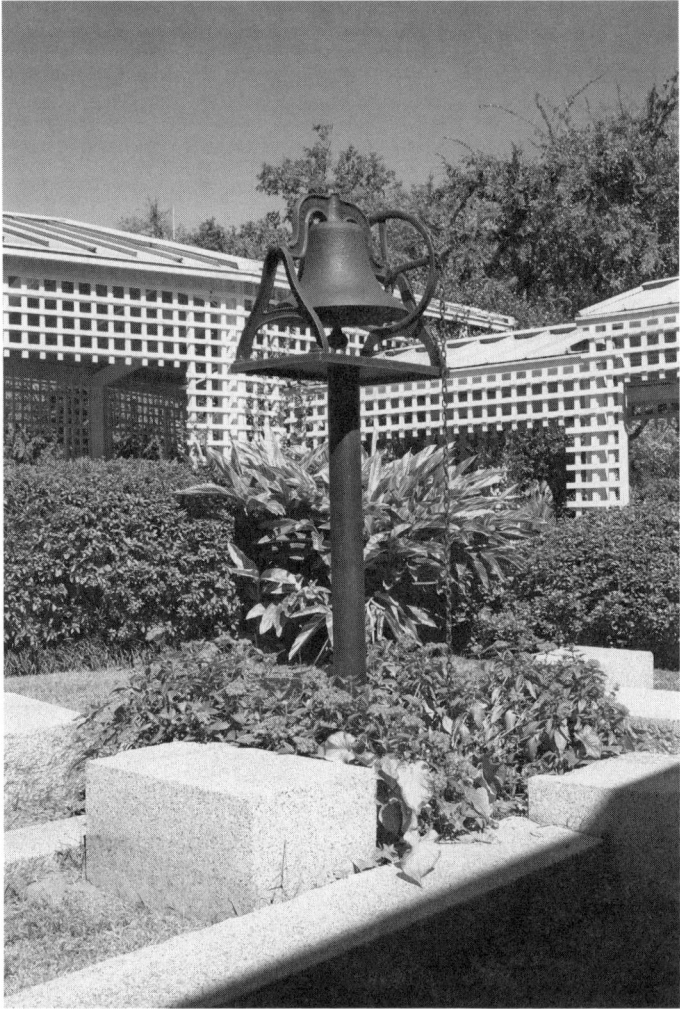

Bell used to call girls to meals.
Photo by Gregory Aycock, Poydras Home Archives

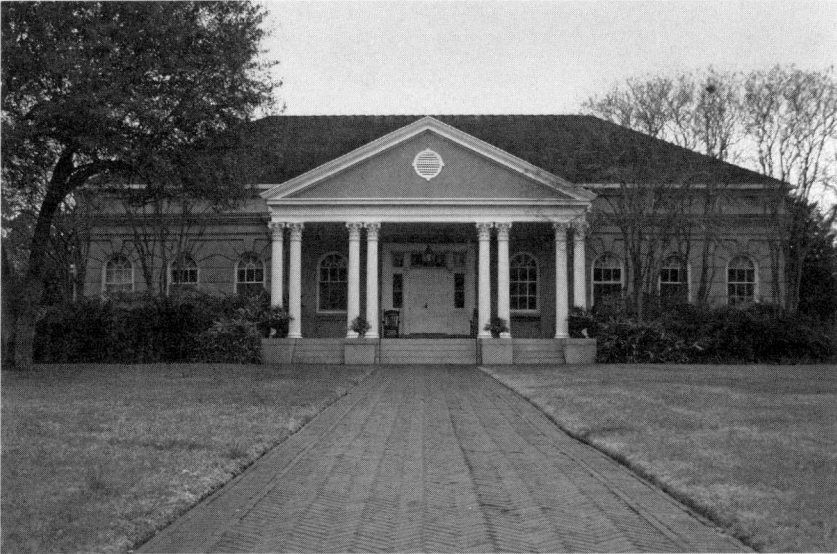

The Poydras Home, after removal of the top two floors.
Photo by Gregory Aycock, 2013, Poydras Home Archives

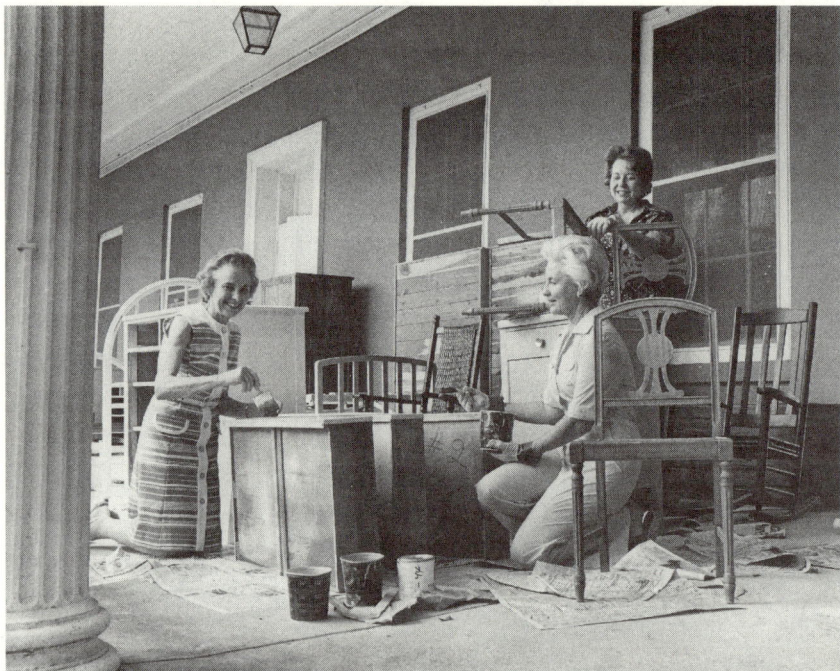

Members of the board of managers working to prepare the Poydras Home
as a residence for elderly women. Pictured left to right are Mrs. H. A. Thompson,
Mrs. Van Law Jones, and Mrs. Philip Holland.
Poydras Home Archives

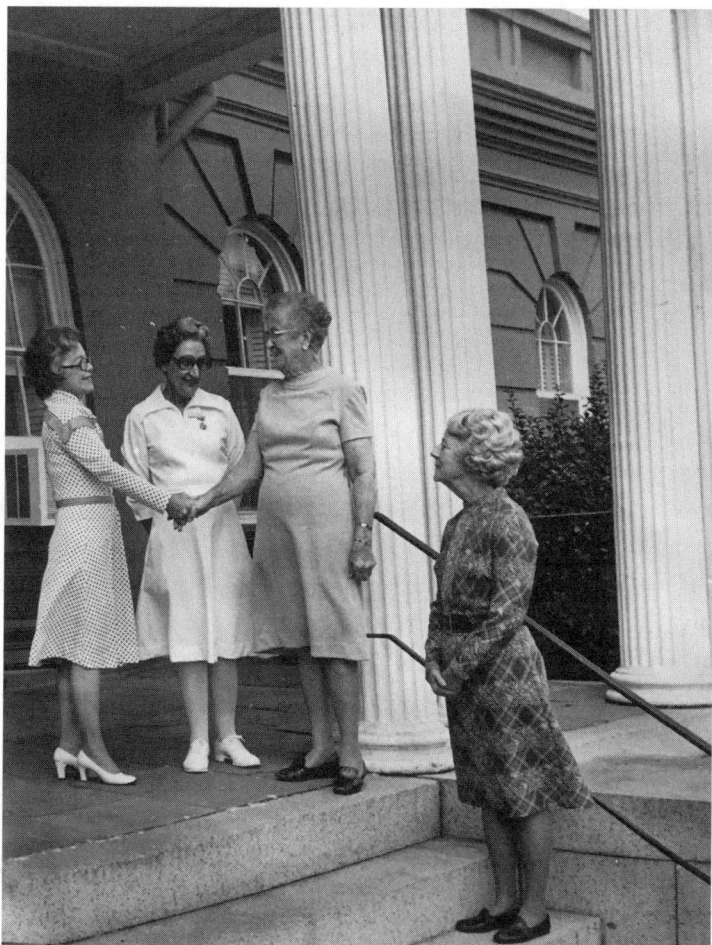

On the veranda at the entrance to the Poydras Home in 1976, Mrs. J. Calvin Williams (*left*), a former board president and chairman of the building committee, along with head nurse Corinna Webb, greets residents Rose Entwisle and Norma Bunting.

New Orleans States-Item, Poydras Home Archives

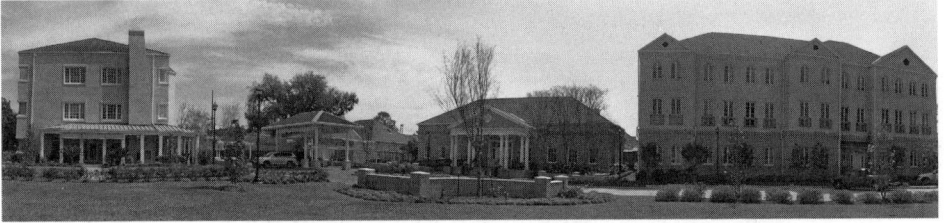

Panoramic view of the Poydras campus today, showing, left to right foreground, Garden House, the original historic building, and Oak House.
Photo by Gregory Aycock, Poydras Home Archives

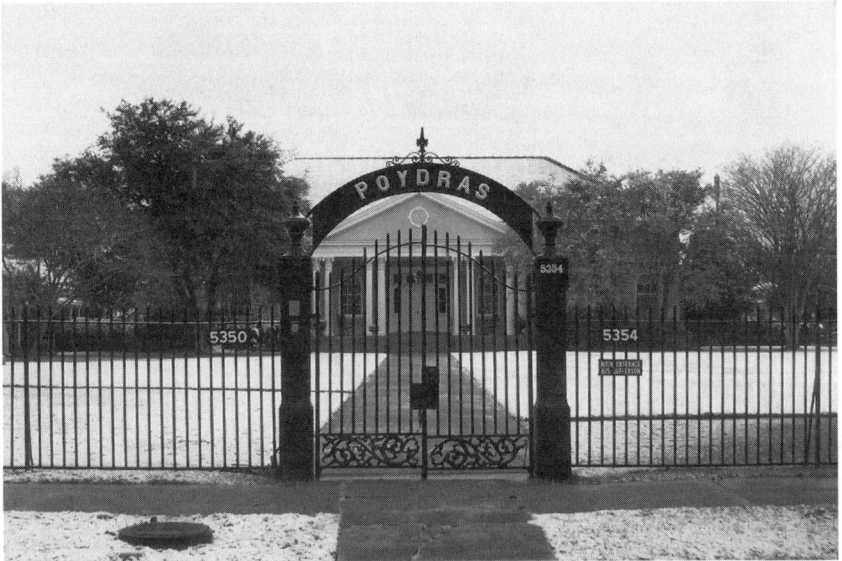

The front gate of the Poydras Home.
Photo by Gregory Aycock, Poydras Home Archives

6

CHALLENGES TO POYDRAS

The Union Army and Reconstruction

The gingham dog went "Bow-wow-wow!"
And the calico cat replied "Mee-ow!"
The air was littered, an hour or so,
With bits of gingham and calico...

The gingham dog and the calico cat
Wallowed this way and tumbled that,
Employing every tooth and claw
In the awfullest way you ever saw—
And, oh! How the gingham and calico flew!

The asylum's records show that it was 1861 when the managers chose religious separatism in their quest for peace at Poydras, seeking to quell religious turmoil at the home by refusing to hire Catholic employees. Ironically, in that year, separatism of a far different kind was rattling the nation, embroiling Americans in a catastrophic civil war and banishing all semblance of peace for years. Beyond the sharp Protestant-Catholic animosity roiling the asylum and much of the country before the war began, an irreconcilable fault line had split Americans into pro-slavery and anti-slavery factions. Although many of the founders of the Female Orphan Society came originally from free states on the Eastern Seaboard, they and the next generation of managers seem to have adapted to the institution of slavery in the Crescent City readily enough. The managers relied on white women to staff their asylum, but, like many in the city, they not uncommonly rented the labor of African slaves. Their incorporated status meant that the independent female managers could draw up contracts stating the wages, the work, and the duration of assignments and, entirely without male intervention, could terminate contracts if their enslaved workers proved unsatisfactory.

On several occasions the minutes mention the hiring of enslaved individuals. The relationships sometimes manifested a personal element, as when the gardener James, an enslaved African hired to cultivate vegetables for the asylum table, felt comfortable asking the ladies for a new hat, to which they readily agreed. In 1825, when the managers learned that his owner planned to sell him, they promptly attempted to buy James, but, uninformed about current prices, they offered a bid nearly 100 percent below his selling price. Three years later, Phoebe Hunter, in her youth a devout Quaker, was charged with enquiring for "a suitable set of slaves" for purchase. After her report, the group authorized her to buy them, but there is no record that she did so. In 1831, the women undertook a serious discussion on "the propriety of purchasing slaves for the use of the institution," but the minutes shed no light on the views presented. Evidently, they could not reach a conclusion on the burning issue of the day.[1]

Though there were "slave pens" located on the upriver side of Canal Street, in the general vicinity of most of the managers' homes, propriety forbade New Orleans women from visiting any of the several slave traders' yards in person; it was widely agreed that they would encounter squalor and misery of a degree that no genteel white woman should witness. The asylum records show Female Orphan Society ownership of one slave, Rachel, whom the managers had purchased as laundress for $400 in 1833; presumably they delegated a local man to carry out the transaction on their behalf. Distressed on an occasion when Rachel showed no remorse after Mrs. Hunter reprimanded her for using insulting language, the managers briskly resolved to sell her at auction if she "persisted in her clamorous and disgusting demeanor." Evidently Rachel bridled her tongue, for two years later, the annual report solemnly noted that "two of the elder inmates" had died in the previous year, mentioning Rachel first, and then Madame Bertoulin, the Frenchwoman who had been seamstress and general housekeeper.[2] Though Bertoulin's suffering from a long and painful illness was recorded, there was no description of Rachel's last days. This omission bears out the conclusions reached by countless historians, who have found that southern white women generally failed to identify with enslaved women or to see that they sometimes shared similar problems.

When mounting sectional conflict reached fever pitch and sundered the Union in 1861, Louisiana seceded with her southern sisters, although southern historian Charles P. Roland judged her "the unlikeliest state of the Deep South to attempt a break with the Union."[3] Much of this unlikely aspect lay rooted with the influential bankers and merchants of New Orleans, whose northern ancestry and economic ties to the cities of the Northeast made them loath to sever their connection to the Union. Many of these men were the fathers and husbands of the Poydras managers. However, the propaganda of militant secessionists dissolved resistance with amazing speed. The Rev. Benjamin Morgan Palmer (1818–1902) of the First Presbyterian Church, labeled by his biographer "the most influential religious figure in the largest, most cosmopolitan southern city,"[4] asserted divine sanction for southern states' secession from the Union in a widely quoted Thanksgiving Day sermon in late 1860. Reverend Palmer referred to Lincoln's election as "that which all men dreaded" and labeled secession "the line of policy which the South has been compelled in self-preservation to adopt." His address, printed and circulated throughout the region, was both a defense of slavery and a vindication of secession, a powerful pro-Confederate manifesto. Many Poydras managers who worshiped in Palmer's congregation each Sunday were soon to feel the iron grip of war on their lives and on their cherished asylum.[5]

The Poydras managers displayed a robustly pro-Confederate spirit upon the outbreak of hostilities. Less than three weeks after the firing on Fort Sumter, they resolved, without dissent, to tender the services of the asylum's sewing department to the local women's aid societies then making clothing for the Confederate army. The asylum's sewing department, in the charge of a head seamstress with assistants, had always taught the older girls to sew and then employed their labor to produce textiles for the asylum and sometimes for sale. Each year, with staff supervision, the girls regularly stitched all necessary clothing as well as household articles like bed linens, tablecloths, and towels. Now, by focusing chiefly on production for the military, by the end of 1861 they had proudly tallied 524 shirts and "drawers" and one hundred coats and pairs of pants made with their hands for the boys in gray. Since every garment made for the military represented a garment not made for the orphans, we may gauge the depth of the board's commitment to the Confederate cause accordingly. Not only did this effort for the Confederate army reduce sewing for the asylum population, it also sacrificed the girls' educations. The annual report for 1861 admitted that progress in school had been poor, noting by way of justification, "our children, in common with persons of every age and sex in our newborn Confederacy, have been diligently employed in making garments for our brave army."[6]

Beyond much-needed clothing, the women in late 1861 shipped a crate of costly medical supplies valued at $500 to a Confederate hospital in Columbus, Georgia. Some managers gave treasure of a more personal nature by sending sons into battle. Minutes from March 1862 note that Mrs. Southmayd was "detained by the departure of her sons for the seat of war," while a month later, Mrs. Luzenberg missed a board meeting because her soldier son was "just returned from the war." January 1864 brought the notation that the latter was "at another post of duty attending the sick bed of her wounded son."[7]

The strategic importance of New Orleans to the Confederacy meant that Union forces would expend the utmost effort to capture the old port city; controlling the Mississippi at its mouth would allow the North to deprive the South of its principal artery. Sadly for the Confederates, the conquest of New Orleans did not require great effort at all. Inadequately defended by two ancient forts downriver and a small force of only 3,000 lightly armed Confederate troops, whose commander withdrew them entirely when the Federal fleet broke through, the city, to the dismay of its disbelieving but still defiant population, fell to David Farragut's gunboats in late April 1862. Bells tolled constantly to warn the population of the imminent arrival of the enemy's forces. A nightmarish scene of confusion unfolded as the last Confederate forces torched warehouses full of cotton and men and women ran about the flaming wharves in panic. When General Benjamin Butler took possession of the city on May 1, it marked the end of civilian government. A succession of Union military authorities would now run the city.

Women of New Orleans proved a particularly sharp thorn in the side of Federal occupation forces because of their notoriously defiant and mocking attitudes. Only two weeks after his arrival, Butler felt compelled to issue his infamous General Order No. 28, mandating that whenever any woman, by word or gesture, showed contempt for U.S. military personnel, she should be "regarded and held liable to be treated as a woman of the town plying her avocation." His implied threat of coarse sexual retribution stirred up hysterical reactions, both locally and far afield, but failed to subdue New Orleans women as he hoped. Still, they sang Confederate airs lustily and played them with spirit upon their parlor instruments; still, they turned scornfully aside, gathering their skirts in disdain when passing Union officers in the streets. Local diarist Julia LeGrand wrote feelingly in her journal, "When I see these officers I do not hide the scorn I feel. I cannot condescend to smile." Deprived of adequate food by the blockade, forbidden to move freely about the city, worried over the safety of absent menfolk, and frequently upset by wild rumors, New Orleans women hardened their hearts toward those who occupied their city. Did Poydras managers and their daughters present a cold and haughty visage to the occupying troops? When LeGrand met the daughters of manager Catherine Pritchard, she approvingly noted their "sublime contempt for the Yankees" and marveled, "They are Philadelphia people. These adopted Southerners are much hotter than we, strange to say."[8]

More than a year after Butler's order, female defiance continued unabated. When a Union officer attempted to disrupt a local church service because the minister refused to pray for the health of President Abraham Lincoln, women of that Episcopal congregation defied the Federals. A bit of local doggerel commemorated the so-called "Battle of St. Paul's":

> Up rose the congregation
> We men were all away
> And our wives and little children
> Alone remained to pray
> But when has the Southern woman
> Before a Yankee quailed?
> And these with tongues undaunted
> The Lincolnites assailed.
> In vain he called his soldiers
> Their darts around him flew
> And the strong men then discovered
> What a woman's tongue can do.[9]

Some months later, in what came to be colloquially called the Battle of the Handkerchiefs, local white women, massed on the levee to see off a transport of Confederate prisoners-of-war, engaged in more defiance by making a tremendous show of waving their handkerchiefs and parasols as a salute of admiration. The commanding general on the scene literally threatened them with force if they did not disperse, but to no avail; their admiring flutterings continued until the boats had sailed out of sight.

In September 1862, Butler issued General Order No. 76, requiring that every New Orleanian, male and female alike, take a loyalty oath by October 1 or be labeled an enemy of the United States. Failure to register would lead to confiscation of the offender's property, which all were required to itemize in detail for purposes of taxation; houses of the nonregistrants were subject to be searched by Union troops at any time. Rumors flew that women who refused the oath would be confined in a large stable and put to work cooking and washing for the Union army. Order No. 76 affected the Poydras board of managers materially, as, only days after its promulgation, three stunned women (Luzenberg, Stringer, and Scriven) resigned their offices in consequence of its requirements. They and their families planned to flee the city rather than take the hated loyalty oath. When Mrs. Stringer sent in her quarterly treasurer's report in October 1862, she appended a terse note explaining that she was "compelled to resign the office from political reasons."[10] The three women appointed to replace them (Newman, Richardson, and Toby) were mentioned in the minutes as "representing loyalty." However, within a few months, all three who resigned their positions were again serving on the board, so obviously they did not take flight and presumably they swore a loyalty oath instead.

By far the conflict's most significant impact upon the Poydras Asylum was financial. A Federal blockade of the city began in late May 1861, but unlike the circumstances just before the War of 1812, when Baratarian freebooters had ignored a trade embargo and smuggled needed goods under the noses of impotent officials, this time there was no brazen pirate Lafitte to bring in scarce goods. The increasingly effective Union blockade choked off imports into New Orleans, created significant scarcities, and quickly drove costs to terrible heights, leading the managers to deplore vastly increased prices of food. They sought to obtain better rates with butchers and bakers by negotiating monthly contracts; they discontinued their practice of having the cook prepare luncheon for them when the board met. Almost from the start, minutes spoke of "the stern necessity of retrenchment," and treasurer Phoebe Laidlaw exhorted the managers to "the most rigid economy . . . to prevent greater embarrassment in our household expenses."[11] The year 1861 saw the paid positions of chaplain and seamstress eliminated and wages cut by one-third for every staff member. The employees allegedly accepted their fate "with hearty good will."[12] Over time, the managers eliminated more workers, eventually even the cook, and brought the "large girls" to labor in their places wherever possible. Meetings routinely began with sober examination of bills—bills for groceries, hay, and feed, cotton cloth, pens for the schoolroom, property insurance, and on and on. They faced choices—to pay the butcher and hold off the baker for one more month, or vice versa? Though financially pinched, they appropriated money to buy an iron safe for secure storage of important papers, indicating their total lack of trust and respect for the enemy, whom they feared capable of burning the asylum. Times were hard, but worse was soon to come.

In 1862, when the Union occupiers "derang[ed] the currency by forbidding the use of Confederate notes," as the society's treasurer phrased it, the managers' cash on hand at a stroke became worthless. Tenants who rented commercial properties from the Female Orphan Society began asking for rent reductions, and as business conditions deteriorated, their requests became clamorous demands. By the end of 1862, only two renters out of six continued to pay for the stores they were still occupying. The managers, certain that some tenants were "perfectly able to pay the amount agreed upon," turned the matter over to their attorney, but court had discontinued regular sessions in the unsettled conditions of war and nothing was done to press their claims. In a delicious bit of turnabout, the women coped with one of their deadbeat tenants, grocer John T. Moore, by buying asylum groceries from him on credit and then neglecting to pay their bill. The revenue stream managed so carefully by the women, ensuring the expansion and prosperity of Poydras, now slowed to a trickle. Even as the number of girls living in the asylum rose, annual income from rents fell by half, plummeting from nearly $24,000 in 1861 to only $13,048 in 1862.[13]

Troubles came in droves, leading the treasurer in early 1863 to lament the "peculiar state of political affairs, which have so sadly destroyed the commerce of the city and ... materially injured the interests of the Society."[14] Indeed, the blockade extinguished once-normal prosperity and impoverished the city. Banks failed; businesses collapsed. Interest on the managers' loan at the Louisiana State Bank came due, but they were unable to pay it. Pledging to pay the bank with the first money that could be procured, they again reduced expenses. Financial belt tightening led the managers to reduce meat consumption at the home to twice weekly. The secretary's records now showed serious discussion over even minute expenses, such as $3 for cornmeal and $7.50 for tea. In a further effort to reduce expenses, they changed their admissions policy. Heretofore, they had allowed each manager, after investigation of circumstances, to order admission of a child on her own authority, but now, in an effort to accept only the neediest children, they required presentation of the facts of each case to the full board of managers when in session at the asylum.

After much consultation, in late 1863 the hard-pressed managers took the unprecedented step of requiring that all adults whom they deemed able to support their children either withdraw them from the Poydras Asylum or begin contributing to their support. In some cases, noncustodial parents bristled at being pressed for payment, as did one man who complained of the women "senshuring me for not paying some thing on my children." Claiming that he knew others of means who dodged payment, he declared, "I am not making the money and aint got it speare" but pledged "if I can I will pay somethin on them." There is no record of the disposition of his case.[15]

As the war limped toward its inevitable close, the managers had occasion to deal both directly and indirectly with Federal authorities, with mixed results. Union officers peremptorily took possession of one of the Female Orphan Society's stores at Poydras and Tchoupitoulas Streets for use as a recruiting office in the occupied city, so upsetting the impotent managers that they contemplated legal action. Then a destructive fire rampaged through the Union Cotton Press, one of their most lucrative rental properties. Rebuilding it burdened the managers with expenses they could ill afford, but which they bore in order to restore essential income. Alas, no sooner was the costly rebuilding accomplished than Alfred Penn, the wealthy businessman who had leased it before the fire, informed the women that Federal authorities had seized it to use as a depot for feed and hay. On Penn's advice, they billed the enemy for the rent, with a pointed reminder that the income sustained orphans. Diarist Julia LeGrand wrote dismissively of the Federal seizure of local properties that "they say rent is to be given ... however, nobody expects payment."[16] Indeed, not until war's end did the Poydras managers realize one cent of payment from the U.S. government for use of this property, and that success came only after they again resorted to the courts. The managers detailed one of their number as liaison with their attorney; she meticulously monitored the progress of the lawsuit and kept the board apprised fully of developments.

In mid-1863, a delegation of four Poydras managers called upon General George Foster Shepley, military governor of Louisiana, hoping to secure his intervention to settle a contested claim against them for drainage costs associated with their lakefront properties at Milneburg. The dyspeptic diarist Julia LeGrand disparaged Shepley, whom she had met, calling him "a deceitful-looking querulous man ... coarse and brutal."[17] Managers Laidlaw, Luzenberg, Richardson, and Toby were evidently able to ignore traits that inflamed LeGrand; fortuitously, the meeting went well and Shepley proved to be a reliable Poydras ally for the remainder of the war. Within the space of the next few months, he personally donated five hundred dollars to the Female Orphan Society, appropriated one thousand dollars to the distressed managers for roof repairs at the home, and promised that the asylum should not be taxed, even as other properties were groaning under newly imposed tax burdens. Shepley was as good as his word, for the minutes note the receipt of an official document from him exempting asylum property from taxation.

The women needed vigilance, however, to parry the relentlessly acquisitive tentacles of the military occupiers. When, despite General Shepley's warm assurances, they received a tax bill in late 1864, they immediately arranged to see General Stephen A. Hurlbut and, eventually, Governor Michael Hahn. Their personal diplomacy at the highest levels of bureaucracy secured the desired outcome when Hahn obligingly suspended the tax. Early in the Union occupation, Colonel Henry Deming, the city's military mayor, had visited the asylum and "could hardly give sufficient praise to our noble institution," according to the managers' notebook. But in 1864, Union general James Bowen cast covetous eyes on the large, three-story asylum, envisioning it as a Union hospital. He demanded to know the exact number of girls in residence and the number whom the structure could reasonably be expected to house, obviously believing that space which the United States Army needed was being underutilized. By this time convinced of the efficacy of the personal approach in dealing with their occupiers, the women delegated one of their number to see Bowen and charged her with informing him of "the extent of the good and charity afforded by the institution." Catharine Pritchard, the manager designated for this mission, pressed her advocacy for the home so effectively that the general abandoned his purpose "and proffered his protection." Ultimately, the managers' relations with Union officials had waxed so warm that, at war's end, General Edward Canby personally intervened to expedite their full recovery of back rent for the Union Cotton Press from the federal government.[18]

In every encounter between officers and women, the power dynamic tilted drastically in favor of the former, but the women of Poydras, proper ladies all, had certain advantages when they faced the occupiers. They ventured forth clad in the highly effective armor of genteel respectability and animated by a spirit of the righteousness of their mission. Annual reports, produced by their secretary and signed by the principal directresses each January, testify eloquently that they viewed their work for the asylum as an almost holy calling. In pursuit of their mission, they never hesitated to press military authorities forthrightly for what they needed and often reminded them bluntly that they provided a home for defenseless young girls, surely society's most vulnerable members. They benefited as well from the nineteenth century's universal acknowledgment of women's role as guardians of the home, members of their sex being peculiarly suited to nurture the young. Attributing to God a direct interest in their work, they saw divine providence in many outcomes. As the dark year of 1864 began, for example, the treasurer, gravely reporting the extent of their heavy indebtedness and urging more stringent economies, closed her report by enjoining all to thank God "that amid the convulsions that have rent asunder our beloved country, you are permitted to assemble around this board . . . your Heavenly Father . . . has not forsaken or forgotten you or your orphan family."[19]

When peace finally came, the weary managers anticipated higher demands upon the asylum to shelter war orphans, but they also felt a cautious optimism that rising commercial rents would ease their pinched situation. The year 1866 saw admissions of orphans of Confederate soldiers whose destitute mothers were unable to provide for them. Increasingly, families in distress turned to Poydras as a temporary shelter for their children. For example, a war widow who lived upstate on the Red River petitioned to have her three daughters admitted for a limited period while she journeyed to "Washington City" to try to reclaim property troops had confiscated during the war.

Unlike many of their fellow southerners, the women of Poydras seemed to be more than ready to bind up the nation's wounds and look forward toward work to be done, rather than backward toward a lost cause. Evidence to support this assertion rests in a small detail tucked among their meticulous records. In early May 1865, they recorded, without comment, an expense of $7.20. This outlay purchased yards of black fabric, with which the managers, erstwhile Confederates all but pragmatic women as well, draped the asylum's massive portico in mourning for Abraham Lincoln.

New Orleans in peacetime was hardly peaceful. In 1866, when Louisiana leaders assembled in the city to draft a new state constitution, hopeful African Americans thronged the pavement outside Mechanics Hall. Their shouts for the right to vote prompted counterdemonstrations by crowds of angry Confederate veterans. Heated voices led to violence; bloodshed and mayhem ruled for hours at the intersection of Common and Dryades Streets. The episode, known as the Mechanics Hall Massacre, left 38 dead and 184 injured, nearly all of them African Americans. A few years later, blood again ran in the streets of New Orleans when white southerners defied the federal government. For a few giddy days after the so-called Battle of Liberty Place, in 1874, the insurrection of whites enjoyed success; hundreds of defiant White Leaguers held the armory and statehouse after clashing with state militia and police loyal to the United States government, but the arrival of federal troops sent by President Ulysses Grant scattered the rebels and restored federal control.

Though not located near these scenes of violence, the Poydras Asylum could not escape the shocks of Reconstruction. Freedmen and freedwomen in New Orleans were keen to take advantage of opportunities to lead better lives after slavery, and this goal often created a fluid workforce. Ill treatment, low wages, and sheer desire for change led to workplace turnover, particularly among African American women, many of whom were at last able to enjoy the roles of wife, mother, and homemaker in homes of their own. Like many other white employers, the Poydras managers found themselves unable to keep a stable domestic staff of washwomen and chambermaids at the asylum, but they were resigned and philosophical about the situation. "In an age of so much restlessness, this [turnover among domestic servants] is to be expected," the secretary wrote in 1871.[20]

The previous year, concern over "restlessness" among the freedpeople in their employ had led the managers to abandon their longstanding belief that the asylum belonged only in the hands of a capable female. Matron Mrs. Kipp, whose excellence they acknowledged, was finding it difficult to "control the outside employees," according to the minutes. The secretary's phrase "outside employees" alluded to the freedmen working as gardeners and day laborers at the asylum, who exhibited a new assertiveness toward white women in their changed postwar circumstances. In response, the managers hired a white married couple. Newcomer Mrs. Sugden replaced faithful Mrs. Kipp as matron, while her husband took charge of repairs, grounds, all of the Poydras rental properties, and all "outside employees." The Sugdens seemed to give complete satisfaction and served for eight years, until an anonymous letter, purporting to be from an orphan, leveled "the most scandalous charges" against both. Although they stoutly denied the charges, which were thought to be too shocking to be included in the minutes, they submitted resignations and the board concluded that "under the circumstances, it was best to sever the connection." The couple's mysterious story came to a tragic end only a few weeks later, in the autumn of 1878, when they were victims of a steamboat explosion as they traveled to their new home up the Red River. Mr. Sugden was killed; his widow was badly burned and lost all her belongings in the disaster. Informed that Mrs. Sugden, bereft and in unremitting pain, needed constant care and was utterly destitute, the women of Poydras brought her back to the home to live out her life.[21]

The economic dislocations of the Reconstruction years markedly diminished Female Orphan Society income. Treasurer Phoebe Laidlaw reported "tenants clamorous for a reduction in rents" since their profits were down. The managers had no recourse but to comply, albeit reluctantly, but when tenants requested repairs or improvements on their buildings, the women refused, "till times improve." Pressed by the hard times, and dismayed that their annual rents had declined by 200 percent, they found it necessary to slash the amount of insurance they carried on properties they owned.[22]

In the turbulent postwar years, new forces controlled Louisiana's government. The executive branch rested in the hands of Governor Henry Clay Warmoth, a Union army veteran and native of Illinois who was all of twenty-six years old, and his African American lieutenant governor, Oscar Dunn, who had been born into slavery in New Orleans. A coterie of non-Louisianians and African Americans dominated the state legislature. The state's 1868 constitutional convention produced a color-blind document for governing Louisiana that mandated equal access for all people in all public accommodations. In such a radical reversal of the prior norm, it must have seemed to most white Louisianians as if the earth were lurching on its very axis. In such parlous times, the Poydras women made a move frankly calculated to prevent the drastic changes abroad in Louisiana from altering the makeup of their board of managers. They amended their constitution to stipulate that future members of the Female Orphan Society would require a two-thirds vote of all current members in order to be allowed to join. Heretofore, any woman who wished to join the society had only to pay her annual subscription of eight dollars, which was later raised to a lifetime fee of one hundred dollars. The secretary noted obliquely that, "in the changed relations of the country," the managers felt "liable at any time to suffer loss by canny and designing persons." Their amendment blocked that possibility. Power would remain in the hands of the old guard; the current membership could reject any woman with a different vision or ideology. If women allied with the new forces in state government, whether carpetbaggers, scalawags, or black-and-tans, should turn a curious eye toward the Poydras Asylum and seek to assist in its management, they would find their entry blocked by those who preferred the *status quo ante bellum*.[23]

Though the female managers had enjoyed a good relationship with city and state governments since the asylum's inception in 1817, they clearly took a dim view of the new governing regime during Reconstruction. During the Reconstruction years, a state senator from Baton Rouge called at the home and left a questionnaire that probed most inquisitively into the institution's finances. The prying lawmaker demanded to know the managers' current expenses and from what sources their operating funds came. The women, however, deigned to make no reply to the gentleman's queries. "As the paper appeared to be without authority, it was decided to take no notice of the same," sniffed the secretary. Accordingly, they provided no information.[24]

We may think of this incident as the proverbial black cloud, no larger than a man's hand, appearing on the far-distant horizon. Like the slight disturbance that expands into a storm of strength and fury, this early inquiry from the state would prove to be a harbinger of intrusions to come. Poydras managers in the twentieth century would find the tendrils of various outside agencies and programs twining in through the gate, and would judge this an unwelcome development. For their first century of existence, the women of the board enjoyed a remarkably free hand in operating their cherished institution exactly as they wished, but, inevitably, that would change.

$$7$$

IN SICKNESS AND IN HEALTH

The Operation of the Poydras Asylum in Its First Hundred Years

> When I was sick and lay a-bed,
> I had two pillows at my head,
> And all my toys beside me lay,
> To keep me happy through the day.

During the asylum's first hundred years, each girl's day featured meals, schoolbooks, and chores. Unfortunately, medicines and mortality often intruded, although the overall picture is emphatically one of health. In this chapter, we will examine daily life at Poydras during its first century.

In October of 1832, a carpenter came to the asylum, bringing with him a badly frightened little girl who appeared to be perhaps ten years of age. He reported that he had found her on the previous evening, huddled on his steps, alone in the dark. Beyond saying that her name was Madeleine, she would not speak at all, though several managers tried gently to elicit a response. They concluded that she was Catholic because, in her fear, she repeatedly made the sign of the cross.

Little Madeleine was almost certainly orphaned by the lethal cholera epidemic ravaging the city in October 1832. Hot, humid New Orleans, poorly drained and surrounded by water, possessed no municipal sewerage disposal system at all until the very end of the nineteenth century; before that time, individuals and businesses handled the need in their own idiosyncratic and mostly inadequate ways. Not surprisingly, the city was a veritable petri dish for the incubation of disease. It takes no great imagination to see that raw sewage not infrequently contaminated the water supply with human fecal material. In that era before scientifically trained public health officials asserted themselves against contagion, periodic outbreaks of deadly diseases flared in the prevailing hot, moist, unsanitary environment; sweeping through the community, pestilence claimed victims at a terrifying rate. Gut-based maladies like typhoid fever, dysentery, and cholera made regular fatal visitations. New Orleans, as a thriving international port, could hardly have avoided the infectious diseases that seemed to arrive on every crowded ship, but had she enjoyed a clean water supply and more adequate sewerage and drainage systems, the death tolls from those diseases would never have reached the alarming figures that history records.

The so-called "Asiatic cholera" spread worldwide as a pandemic in 1832, stalking victims across the globe from east to west. After extinguishing hundreds of thousands of lives in India in the 1820s, the disease spread to Russia in 1831, from there to central Europe, and then on to London and Paris. By the summer of 1832, Quebec and Montreal had experienced an outbreak, and within days, cholera had hitchhiked to New York City, news that sent perhaps one hundred thousand New Yorkers, 40 percent of the city's population, in panicky flight to the presumably healthier countryside. By fall of 1832, the pestilence had arrived in New Orleans.

Contributing significantly to the horror being felt was the grim fact that, after a sudden onset of dramatic and alarming symptoms, death often came with stunning rapidity. Cholera was an acute infectious disease, characterized by vomiting, painful cramps, and intensely profuse, watery diarrhea. The cholera bacillus, taking up residence in the small intestine, effectively ended absorption of liquids, multiplied wildly, and caused the body to dehydrate itself severely and sometimes fatally within a matter of hours. The pitiable child Madeleine may have been witness to the demise of one or both parents from this killer. From what we know of the course of this disease, on a day in late October 1832, she might well have received porridge and milk from a smiling, seemingly healthy mother at breakfast, only to be orphaned by sundown. Her mother may have called out to her for assistance as her body produced ten to twenty liters of diarrhea, draining all hydration from her body, leaving her skin cold and bluish-gray, her pulse rapid and weak, and her blood pressure dangerously low. Within a matter of only a few hours, she might have sunk into an unconsciousness from which she never emerged. It is little wonder that the stricken child sat dazed and silent, alone in the darkness, before the kindly carpenter found her.

Though today cholera typically responds quickly and well to simple oral or intravenous rehydration, antebellum doctors' approaches to case management illustrated the thinking characteristic of the age of "heroic medicine," when physicians attempted to produce in their patients a strong and visible reaction to the drug or treatment being administered as "proof" that their services merited compensation. Sufferers in the 1830s were bled until they fainted, dosed with poisonous mercury until they salivated profusely, or burned until blisters appeared on their skin. A Louisiana doctor remarked jovially that he had drawn off enough blood during the cholera epidemic to float the steamboat *General Jackson*. Worst of all, there was no understanding of the transmission of this disease. Some blamed "miasmas," or bad air; a few suspected the water supply, but without proof. Many targeted the immigrant population then surging into the Crescent City from Ireland and Germany, observing smugly that filth, poverty, and vice were the causative agents.

At the time of the 1832 cholera epidemic, New York City boasted a population more than four times greater than that of New Orleans. Though the disease claimed over 3,000 lives in New York, that figure seems low if compared with the death toll of approximately 4,300 lives when cholera rampaged through the less populated New Orleans in a period of about one month, taking perhaps 20 percent of the population still in residence. At the first November board meeting of that year, only Phoebe Hunter and Phoebe Laidlaw attended; all the others were away "in consequence of prevalence of cholera." Although board attendance was feeble at the height of the fearful epidemic, the managers admitted upwards of twenty orphaned girls during that sickly season. Remarkably, there were no deaths from cholera at the Poydras Asylum in 1832. The managers gave prayerful thanks to the Almighty for his mercy, and direct thanks to the staff for their gentle and capable nursing of sick girls.

The report of Poydras physician Dr. J. Rhodes to a regional medical journal provides insight into the asylum's experience with the later severe cholera epidemic of 1849. Although, in that year, no cases of the disease developed at the Poydras Asylum for the first two months of the epidemic's siege on the city, in late February 1849, unmistakable symptoms began to appear among the girls. Over the next three weeks, some sixty cases developed at Poydras, and ten of them were fatal. Dr. Rhodes leaves us with a vivid description of the disease's distressing effects on the girls.

> The desire of drink was in every case very urgent, the fluid seldom retained, being thrown up almost immediately with great force; still the little sufferers continued their plaintive cry for *water, water* (in the fatal cases) till the last moment of articulation.
>
> The features became so altered, as the symptoms of collapse came on, and in many cases they came on with astonishing rapidity, that it was almost impossible to recognize the most familiar face, with its sunken eye and livid expression. As the stage of collapse progressed, the skin became icy cold, small, feeble pulse, cold breath and tongue.... Vomiting and purging continued with but few exceptions till the last moment, the intelligence remaining good till death closed the scene.[1]

Though the powerful cholera epidemics of 1832 and 1849 wracked New Orleans particularly hard, the Poydras managers had from the very beginning regularly faced serious illness among their charges and themselves. An examination of the group's minutes shows that in their first year of operation, they canceled all meetings for over four months because of what they called "the present alarming epidemic," and again in 1818, they held no meetings for five months for the same reason. Following the pattern of settlers from the Eastern Seaboard, most Poydras managers of the early years absented themselves from the city when "the sickly season" descended in midsummer, annually fleeing the most feared of all diseases.[2]

That disease was yellow fever, a dreaded malady colloquially called "Bronze John" and "Yellow Jack" by citizens who perhaps hoped to tame its ferocity by domesticating the pestilence with familiar nicknames. Again, as with cholera, medical practitioners did not understand transmission of this disease and generally blamed bad night air emanating from swampy settings rather than bites from infected mosquitoes. Also as with cholera, they blamed immigrants, citing filth and poverty as factors. In this case, they were correct, but not for the reasoning they used. Most native New Orleanians had developed immunity after light infections in childhood, but newcomers were highly susceptible to the virus. Epidemics flared when carrier mosquitoes found a large

population of vulnerable individuals, the newly arrived foreigners. Historian
Jo Ann Carrigan, noting these facts, observed that the pattern of epidemics
served to reinforce the nativism of many New Orleanians.

Yellow fever's initial indiscriminant symptoms included chills, muscle
aches, and an elevated temperature, but for many, the disease progressed to
the next and lethal stage involving high fever, liver damage, and severe internal bleeding. Liver malfunction led to jaundice, thus the name "yellow fever,"
but many called the illness "the black vomit" because of the most alarming
effect of this hemorrhagic fever. As with cholera, treatment was dramatic without being effective; physicians bled patients copiously through venesection or
leeching, dosed them with calomel, opium, and quinine, and not infrequently
applied blistering agents. Occasionally, as John Duffy, the premier historian
of Louisiana medicine observed drily, "in a fine demonstration of man over
medicine, the patient survived."[3]

New Orleans death rates from yellow fever hovered around 20 percent
through the antebellum years. Duffy notes that, at a conservative estimate,
in twelve of the thirty-five years between 1825 and 1860, over one thousand
individuals died of yellow fever in New Orleans annually. In the worst years,
the mortality figures were simply shocking. Yellow fever claimed over 1,500
in 1841 and again in 1843; in 1847, its death toll numbered 2,700. In the sto-
ried epidemic of 1853, the disease took a horrifying 9,000 lives in New Orleans; it tallied at least 2,500 in each of the next two years, and killed 5,000 in
1858. When weighing these astounding numbers, one must also consider that
roughly one-third of the city's population fled at the first sign of yellow fever
and stayed away until the pestilence ebbed, so the figures represent deaths
among a significantly flight-reduced citizenry.

In 1820, nearly two dozen Poydras girls, about 40 percent of the residents,
had "the fever" during the summer months, but, remarkably, all recovered.
Three years later, the managers admitted forty-six "unhappy beings" orphaned
when yellow fever killed their parents. Although earlier allusions to "the epidemic which infected the city" or "that dreadful epidemic" almost certainly
referred to yellow fever, the minutes' first mention of yellow fever by name
comes in 1824, when, at the mayor's request, the women took in fourteen
more girls orphaned by the disease. Staff members, too, contracted the deadly
fever. Twenty-two-year-old Sister Lorentia lingered for a week before suc-

cumbing in 1835, "tranquil and perfectly resigned," according to the minutes, while tutoress Mrs. Montgomery recovered, surviving both the fever and a treatment of leeching.[4]

Yellow fever was a regular caller at the asylum during the hot months, but fatalities were notably rare; in 1837, for example, over 50 percent of the 124 resident girls fell ill with yellow fever, yet only one child died. During the noted epidemic year of 1853, fifty-three of the 119 Poydras girls fell ill of yellow fever, with eight fatalities. In its forty-three years of operation between 1817 and 1860, extant records indicate a total of 203 girls' deaths, from all causes—an average of not quite five deaths per year.

The yellow fever scourge of 1853, said by John Duffy to have been the worst epidemic ever to strike New Orleans, tested the institution's tradition of pulling together in time of crisis as never before. Bronze John invaded the asylum in August and produced fifty-one cases in fifty-nine days, most of them severe. The matron fell so ill that the managers took the unusual step of hiring a trained nurse to care for her. But beyond that one extra nurse, they employed only a "watcher" for two nights and an extra laundress for six days; otherwise, regular staff and the girls themselves tended the delirious patients, washed the dirtied bedclothes, and made countless trips for cool compresses, fresh water, and ice during a two-month siege of sickness. In the stricken city around them, every able-bodied citizen's efforts centered on caring for the sick or disposing of the dead. The stench of decomposing corpses wafted on each hot breeze as drunken laborers struggled unsuccessfully to dig wet graves quickly enough, throwing bodies into common burial trenches and layering them with quicklime. Adding a surreal and typically unscientific note of sound and fury were the booming cannons, fired in hopes of dissipating the unhealthy "miasma," and the eerie glare of flames and fingers of black smoke, rising skyward as barrels of tar were burned in a fruitless effort to banish the contagion.

Against this backdrop of crisis, the designated visiting committee of managers called regularly at the asylum; their reports, written by Phoebe Laidlaw, give a clearly etched portrait of the difficult days. At the end of August 1853, she noted four deaths, fourteen girls convalescing, and five still gravely ill, plus the matron who was "not out of danger." All the managers who had not fled the city had been constant visitors, which experience enabled them to evaluate and praise the work of all at Poydras. "In the midst of this calamity," Laidlaw wrote, "your committee feel there is much for which to be grateful, to thank God and take courage." A month later, Laidlaw's tone was almost jubilant as she noted no new cases in the past three days and recoveries proceeding apace, a welcome respite from crisis that allowed time to have the infirmary "thoroughly cleansed," probably with vinegar. In the manner of a military commander writing commendations of troops who will be decorated for their heroic exploits, Laidlaw wrote glowingly of the veteran housekeeper whose "fire has been constant and nourishment for the sick always ready," of the head of the infirmary who stayed so "faithful and true" that there was not a single case of relapse even though six members of her own family fell ill, of the overburdened washers who "with much additional work" labored "with a willing cheerfulness." Her account made space for the humblest contributions as she noted the work of the "little errand goers . . . who through heat or rain, day or night," had fetched needed supplies.[5]

Laidlaw wrote at length of longtime teacher Caroline Bowers, who, though in mourning for her own daughter who succumbed to the disease, merited "the name of the Orphans' Friend" for her steady efforts to soothe badly frightened children during the worst of the epidemic. Insisting on God's love for little children and his ability to hear heartfelt prayers, Bowers urged the shaken girls to pray. She reported to a gratified Laidlaw what she had overheard. "I do not feel a bit afraid of the fever now," said one orphan. "I did as Mrs. Bowers told me and kneeled down by my bed and prayed so hard . . . God heard me." Laidlaw, powerfully affected by Bowers's rendition of the trusting little girls' conversation, approvingly saw in it "unmistakable evidence of the Christian influence pervading, without ostentation, our Institution." In reflecting on their trial during the epidemic, a well-pleased Laidlaw divined proof that the managers' efforts were succeeding in shaping girls who showed "love for each other, unselfishness, cheerful performance of duty and a steadfast looking to God for protection from all danger."[6]

During another serious epidemic of yellow fever in 1878, the devout managers were quick to credit divine intervention as well as science when the asylum was spared. "Every means was used with powerful disinfectants & a strict quarantine enforced & prayer offered to Him who could save us. It was heard, and although the pestilence raged all around us, it was kept from us.

One death occurred, feared at first to be fever, but proved congestion and to-day we would record our gratitude with grateful hearts."[7]

Through the nineteenth century, the asylum endured outbreaks of various contagions. In addition to cholera and yellow fever, the minutes mention multiple cases of whooping cough, measles, dysentery, smallpox, scarlet fever, and diphtheria, serious diseases whose victims often required medical attention. Doctors' annual reports also mention maladies unknown today: "scald head," "whitlow," "marasmus," and "putrid sore throat," for example. In the earliest years, the institution featured a "sickroom," but by 1832, the year of the devastating cholera epidemic, minutes refer to "the infirmary," a space stocked with medicines, well equipped for care of the sick, and used for no other purpose. Even before the asylum opened its doors in 1817, the women had secured the professional services of a local doctor, whom manager Mrs. N. K. Wolstoncraft approached, successfully, about donating his time. Soon, however, they offered an annual stipend to each individual who served as house physician. These doctors usually served for a few years before tendering a resignation, the demands on their time no doubt being considerable in managing the health of upwards of one hundred girls.

For some years, Dr. Charles A. Luzenberg was the Poydras physician; his wife Mary Fort Luzenberg served nearly fifty years on the board of managers. Born in Vienna, educated in Europe, and fluent in French and English, Luzenberg ranked among the leading medical men in New Orleans in the 1830s and 1840s. One of the seven original faculty members at the Medical College of Louisiana, he pioneered in vascular surgery and use of anesthesia in New Orleans, operated a well-regarded private hospital called the Franklin Infirmary, and served as first president of the city's Medico-Chirurgical Society. He was one of the eight prominent physicians whom the managers consulted when the asylum suffered an outbreak of an unidentified malady in 1834. Necessitating the complicated removal of the entire population to other quarters for three months, that illness was called "an ascorbic affection" by the medical panel. Luzenberg also attended girls during outbreaks of "ophthalmia," a serious inflammation of the eyes that could lead to blindness, and oversaw quarantine arrangements for the sick children. It was often his policy to prescribe removal to the country for sick girls, for a "change of air." The minutes not infrequently mentioned him by name in order to praise his kind attentions during epidemics.

However, in 1838, scandal darkened Luzenberg's name and rocked the medical establishment of the city. Judged by John Duffy to have been "a forceful and aggressive personality, a man of strong friendships and bitter enmities," Luzenberg, whose fortuitous marriage to a wealthy widow had enhanced both his status and his fortune, was undeniably a self-promoter and publicity hound.[8] His appetite for headlines proved his downfall when an investigating committee of three physicians (all members of the local medical society, of which he was also a member) ruled that he had knowingly abetted a local newspaper reporter in greatly inflating an account of an unremarkable cataract operation he performed on an elderly Seminole woman. When the society charged him with professional misconduct for allowing or, more likely, encouraging a false report of his surgery to be published, he declined their invitation to appear and explain himself. Instead, he sent what his colleagues called "an offensive and ungentlemanly communication" and resigned from the medical society.

Subsequent events indicate that in all likelihood the ill feeling between Luzenberg and colleagues had deeper roots than mere disagreement over his Seminole cataract case. The medical society, upon receipt of Luzenberg's tantrum on paper, declined to accept his resignation and instead expelled him, taking the further and highly unusual step of ordering that a summary of the case be sent to all medical societies and medical journals in the country. When the blackballed doctor took to the local papers to attack the integrity of the medical society's members, they turned their full wrath upon him, excoriating Luzenberg in print as "a man of ordinary capacity, very little improved by education and study," who had been forced off the medical college faculty by colleagues who deplored "his mendacity, ignorance, presumption, and ill-breeding."[9] In a pamphlet dedicated to damning Luzenberg for all his shortcomings, the local physicians did not hesitate to include a sworn statement from a doctor who averred that Luzenberg, in preparing for a duel with another doctor whom he had insulted, had used cadavers at Charity Hospital for target practice, suspending the dead bodies with chains while he shot at them with his pistol. The cadavers he mutilated were allegedly people who had died while under his care at Charity. Amazingly, Luzenberg did not deny this appalling charge. Instead, he petulantly flung invitations to duel at three separate physicians. All coolly demurred, one remarking, "The infamy which has been stamped upon Dr. Luzenberg's character cannot and shall not be washed away in my own blood."[10]

Yet Dr. Luzenberg had defenders in some quarters; for example, the New Orleans Bee (L'Abeille) called the charges against him "indecente, unjust, grossière."[11] Historians agree that, at the remove of so many years, it is difficult to know which side was right, because the Luzenberg case split the medical community, with prominent physicians on both sides. The women of Poydras stoutly maintained their faith in the controversial doctor, who was after all married to their friend and fellow manager. The board's minutes contain no record of dissension nor even of a discussion on the wisdom of retaining his services, and the dueling doctor continued his association with the asylum until his death in 1848.

Over the years, various doctors attended to Poydras children, and in general, the managers found themselves well pleased with their service. During the First World War, however, managers turned to female caregivers after becoming dissatisfied with the inadequate attentions and high-handed attitude of their male staff physician. Rather than make a scheduled house call at Poydras, the busy Dr. Hamilton Jones had his "office girl" telephone to ask about the condition of several sick children. The assistant relayed the cavalier doctor's instructions that, should medical attention be necessary, Poydras should send for another physician, whom Dr. Jones had selected without input from the managers and, moreover, an individual whom they did not care for. Offended at what they perceived as his arrogance, the Poydras managers sent the errant doctor a brusque note to say that they no longer required his services. Jones, obviously hoping to keep his Poydras position and his income from it, wrote that he was "very much surprised" at their message, but the deed was done. They retained the celebrated Dr. Sara T. Mayo, with agreement that she would be consulting physician at no charge, with her associate Dr. Etta Pearl McCormick the regular attending physician for the asylum. This turn to women started a trend; two months later, they replaced their male dentist with a woman, Dr. Haidee Guthrie.[12]

In October 1918, the lethal influenza epidemic then sweeping the nation afflicted very nearly every resident in the asylum. Dr. McCormick faithfully attended the dozens of stricken girls until she too was taken with the disease. Dr. Mayo then attended in her stead until the contagion waned in November. Though nearly everyone in the asylum, both girls and staff, lay ill for a time, there were no deaths. As with the nineteenth-century epidemics, the kind and steadfast attention of healthy girls for the ill was instrumental in coping with the crisis. Though medicine could do little for this viral infection, the girls themselves, under supervision of the adults, made sure that no sick girl lacked for blankets, broth, water, or cold compresses for fever. In December the board personally thanked thirteen "large girls" for their special service as nurses and, when they left the boardroom, voted to give each a special Christmas gift. The fact that there were no fatalities whatever at Poydras, despite 106 cases of influenza, is all the more remarkable when one considers that the influenza/pneumonia fatality rate in New Orleans in 1918 exceeded that of every major city in the United States.[13]

To what is this generally benign outcome due, decade after decade? It is difficult to know precisely whose agency to credit when evaluating the generally favorable statistics on death rates at the Poydras Asylum. The Poydras managers forthrightly credited the women of their resident staff with being "watchful and benevolent guardians" of the sick girls in their care. They directed praise to their attending physicians, thanking them for their skillful attentions during "a season of unexampled peril and fatigue." In an age before the advent of modern pharmaceuticals, physicians could offer nothing that cured a sufferer of cholera, yellow fever, or influenza, although they frequently tried, with a frightening array of futile approaches. But the records are silent about the administering of any "heroic" remedies to the Poydras girls, whether because the managers did not choose to pay for bleeding, blistering, and calomel, or because they felt such treatments were not appropriate for children. We may assume that attending physicians generally "did no harm" at Poydras, a situation that surely contributed to survival.[14]

Secondly, unlike much of the population of New Orleans, most Poydras girls enjoyed a level of basic good health that fortified them to withstand illness. Although the diet prepared for the girls certainly waxed and waned in quantity and quality over the years, they ate adequate meals of reasonably good quality three times every day. Because their level of nutrition almost certainly exceeded that of the city's poor, they faced disease in a more robust state of health than many New Orleanians.[15] Moreover, after 1857, when the managers built a new orphanage in a bucolic location upriver from the city, they lived in a notably healthy site away from the filth of urban New Orleans. The first asylum had occupied unhealthy low ground that drained poorly, a perfect breeding spot for disease-carrying mosquitoes. As the American, or upriver, commercial sector of New Orleans experienced a tremendous growth spurt in the antebellum period, the teeming city encroached upon the original orphanage site, once the location of Julien Poydras's tranquil plantation. The resultant urban squalor surrounded the asylum; mucky ditches reeking with the contents of countless slop jars and overflowing after each heavy rainfall ran alongside unpaved streets spotted with horse droppings and buzzing with flies, and these sources of pestilence drained into the original home's grounds.

In the aftermath of a season of yellow fever in 1847, before the asylum moved to its more rural location, the society's secretary commented gratefully in her annual report that "an unusual degree of health was enjoyed within these walls, while beyond its precincts unexampled suffering and mortality prevailed." Noting that the year's epidemic had claimed victims of high and low station, she observed that "this humble and helpless family were guarded and safely conducted thro' this season of peril unscathed by the blighting sickness which surrounded them."[16] Yet, despite a fortunate outcome in that year, the annual death rate among the girls in the original asylum location was 10 percent or higher for fully half of the years for which figures are available.

When the managers moved the children to the suburb of Rickerville in 1857, leaving the city of New Orleans four miles behind and taking up life "in the country," tangible benefits ensued. Life in the spacious new building on ample, well-drained grounds placed the children in a much more healthful situation. Having the girls housed, fed, and educated in one healthy place, sequestered on the asylum grounds and rarely allowed to venture outside its gates, isolated them to a degree from exposure to some contagions. After the change of location in 1856, the asylum's mortality rate was impressively low, never again exceeding 3 percent of the institution's population in any year, with the one exception of 8 percent in 1858, which was a yellow fever epidemic year. In fact, deaths at the asylum declined steadily after the move, and in many years, there were no fatalities among the girls, though epidemics continued to afflict New Orleans.

Other factors notwithstanding, fairness compels one to emphasize that the children themselves gave brave and steadfast service through bouts of sickness. Some uncomplainingly ran errands for ice and medicines; others ("large girls") steadily shouldered bedside nursing duties. Handwritten pages in crumbling ledger books tell the story of the kind service of children for their friends. The managers often found it appropriate to recognize the girls for unselfish and outstanding service. For example, when Frederica Bauer died "after great suffering," they presented a silver thimble to Caroline Newman, noting that she had been "particularly kind and attentive" to Frederica during her illness. Diligent attention to the sick earned Eliza Hill "a new frock." When the asylum saw the end of a month-long measles epidemic that had sickened sixty-three girls, with four fatalities, the managers awarded a tucking comb (an ornamental device for holding the hair in place) and a pair of shoes to each of three girls who had shown "exemplary conduct during the sickness in the institution." A dozen others earned new gloves.[17]

In an intact home, a mother tended to her sick child, providing important physical comforts like soft pillows, clean linens, fresh water, and adequate meals. She met her loved one's emotional needs during an illness, soothing and calming a fretful or frightened child. Although they lived in a large institution, sick children at Poydras did not lack for steady, attentive bedside care. Healthy girls nursed the sick, hour after hour and day after day. Unfailingly attentive nursing care, often provided by the girls themselves under caring and intelligent adult supervision, is probably the most important factor in explaining the notably low death rates that prevailed at the Poydras Home. Giving material comfort and the intangibles of attention and affection, motherless girls mothered each other.

Babies at Poydras constitute the one glaring exception to the overall record of good health. The managers of the Poydras Asylum were never inclined to operate a full-fledged baby nursery in their institution. Instead, like most orphan asylums of the nineteenth century, they maintained age limits for admission and preferred to accept no child who was not yet weaned. Of course, exceptions arose. For example, on a cold February morning in 1843, staff at the asylum discovered an infant about four months old suspended from their fence rail in a basket. Her pleading mother had left a note imploring the "most honored ladies" to "be merciful to an unfortunate being who solicits your protection for her child, who has given all she had for its nurture and is destitute of all means ... in these hard times." They accepted the little foundling, but, sadly, she fell victim to smallpox the next month, not strong enough to recover as the other five asylum sufferers did.[18]

Generally, in cases involving very young babies, the managers much preferred to pay the mother a small stipend to help her to keep a child who was still nursing, but if that could not be arranged, they did admit infants, though reluctantly. Asylums that accepted babies had much higher mortality rates than those that did not. Historian Linda Gordon reports that in the late nineteenth century, a stunning asylum death rate of over 90 percent for children under three years of age was "not uncommon," in part attributable to the seriously poor health of the little ones when they arrived and in part due to the hazards then involved in bottle feeding. No understanding of "germ theory," failure to sterilize bottles, and an often-adulterated milk supply combined to write a death sentence for many motherless babies, most often in summer's heat.[19]

The Poydras managers grieved the loss of babies entrusted to their care, as the emotion in this secretary's report from 1869 shows: "The Angel of Death has been permitted twice to enter our nursery, and translate two of our little ones, whom it was our pleasure to cherish. Emma Rose, aged 16 months died June 17 and Elizabeth Beatty, aged 9 months, July 1, just two weeks apart. They were delicate children when they were entered, half orphans, and we hoped that good food and nursing would have effected a change but the Giver of Life thought otherwise and we bow to the supremacy of His Will."[20]

A few months later, the women still felt the pain of the babies' death. "The Board has well nigh come to the conclusion to take no child from the breast," the secretary recorded, observing, "Our experience on this point has been rather painful. Notwithstanding all our care of the few infants committed to us, two has [sic] been transferred to a better world." Yet, time and again, cases tugged their heartstrings and they were prevailed upon to take in an infant. Among others, they cared for foundlings whom they named Emma Poydras and Julia Poydras. Both died. Alas, the outcome often was not good. In 1872, there were three deaths, all infants, whom they chose to remember as the Good Shepherd's "little lambs" [who] "shall hunger no more, and the piteous wail, issuing from physical causes, which medical skill could not remove, will be forever hushed in the songs of Heaven." Again in 1916, minutes noted the death of "little Dorothy Calecas, aged 17 months [who] was admitted four weeks ago, a delicate babe who had never been well," and observed that "many years have past [sic] since Death has entered this home." Of necessity, the managers purchased plots in the Lafayette Cemetery on Washington Avenue. Their chosen inscription for the communal tombstone read "Poydras Home Rest."[21]

Despite this recital of illnesses and occasional deaths, the great majority of children at Poydras enjoyed good health. Beyond providing the girls with adequate health care and proper nutrition, the managers also guaranteed mental nourishment. Young children remained in the nursery for supervised play until age six, at which time they progressed into the large schoolroom, where the curriculum included standard subjects of a good primary education. Pedagogical conditions at Poydras were far from ideal, however, as scholars of all ages mingled and recited in close proximity. When exigencies of the asylum demanded the labor of "large girls," they were pulled from class in order to pitch in with domestic duties. Though teachers' responsibilities were many, their pay was low, and in consequence, turnover was fairly high.

In 1891, the board of managers at last elected to close the on-campus school and send Poydras girls to the public schools of New Orleans. Accordingly, each morning, an employee walked the youngsters to McDonogh #7, a tall, dark brick structure located at Milan and Chestnut Streets, and another employee returned to shepherd them home each afternoon. Though the board members followed a policy of withdrawing girls from McDonogh when they turned fourteen unless they displayed scholastic aptitude, they consistently rejected requests from girls who wished to end their schooling before that point. Poydras girls were thus part of an important minority, namely, the 39 percent of youngsters of school age who were actually enrolled in New Orleans schools at the turn of the twentieth century. Moreover, managers actively encouraged good scholars to attend high school. Advancement required passing an entrance exam, and minutes note with pride each instance of success on that count. Managers regularly heard from the school committee about girls' report cards, noted examples of excellence and failure, and discussed teachers' comments and concerns. As needed, they met with the children's teachers.

The smooth operation of the home relied upon the unpaid women of the board, who devoted much time to its management. In twos and threes, they staffed committees for overseeing admissions, housekeeping, garden and livestock, sewing, purchasing, school, and health. No other body had greater importance than the visiting committee, charged with maintaining a regular physical presence at the home. Throughout the nineteenth century, at least twice weekly, visiting managers spent the better part of the day at the asylum, interacting and observing. Managers' visits in the summer of 1858 reveal the sort of detail they observed. "Dinner nicely cooked in abundance. Children orderly and well-behaved," their notes recorded.[22] They visited the schoolroom, where they examined the writing books and heard spelling and arithmetic; the infirmary, where they took note of the number of sick girls, what the nurse reported about them, and when the doctor would come; and the sewing room, where they inventoried garments made and commented approvingly about the small neat stitches the girls employed. These painstaking visits allowed them to gauge the mood of the staff, whether cheerful or aggrieved. If children were being given overly heavy workloads, they observed it and acted to remedy the situation. Women rotated among the committees approximately every two months, allowing every board member to learn all aspects of their endeavor.

Nineteenth-century managers were quick to reprimand negligent employees and to dismiss those found guilty of serious deficiencies. Use of coarse language and abuse or neglect of the girls drew the swiftest, most severe responses. In 1840, more in sorrow than in anger, they sternly reprimanded their head seamstress, Miss Bertoulin, noting that they had learned "with *deep, very deep* feelings of regret" that she had spoken in an unseemly manner to some of the children. Her intemperate language posed a threat to the refuge from immorality they intended to provide for the girls and introduced a sordid element from which they strove to guard those in their custody.

> You said to one she was fit only to be dressed in sailor's clothes and dance with the *men* in the *sailors' boarding house*. This institution has been established not only as a present home for destitute youth, but that the influ-

ence of pure morals and gentle affections inculcated and fostered here may exercise their controlling influences hereafter upon these poor orphans, when they are sent forth. . . . The managers therefore particularly request that all allusions however remote to subjects having an opposite tendency, should never be made within the walls of the Poydras Asylum. The children must look to the ladies placed over them for *models,* and the managers expect those ladies will at all times be very guarded in their expressions . . . before the children of the institution.[23]

They dismissed a nurse for her excessive absences and neglect of sick children. They promptly fired the matron Mrs. Henry when they learned to their horror that, during the cholera epidemic of 1849, she had punished children by shutting them up alone in "the burial room" where they laid out corpses. (This information "excited the Managers extremely," the minutes noted.) Henry's refusal to help in the infirmary during the crisis also contributed to their decision. "You were required in cases of immergency [*sic*] to assist in the night watches, and render such aid as might be expected *from a mother,*" they reminded Henry in her dismissal notice. "Your fears have deterred you from entering the infirmary."[24]

Despite the managers' earnest assumption that the matron should have acted as "a mother," in spite of their sincere efforts to create a "home" for indigent or neglected girls, no one could have confused life at the asylum with life in a genuine home. Regimentation of necessity characterized Poydras in the nineteenth century. In the earliest years, the children rose at five in warm weather, at six the other half of the year. (The hour for rising was gradually modified to a later time.) They assembled in the schoolroom for roll call, then were dismissed to the washroom, where the younger girls were "combed" by an attendant. Then, neatly dressed, with shoes tied, they were to "walk orderly" to breakfast. They spent mornings in the schoolroom, ate dinner at 12:30, and returned to classes or domestic chores at two. After an early light supper, the younger children went to bed at dark; the older ones could study or amuse themselves before retiring by nine. Saturdays found the girls occupied in cleaning and scrubbing, and Sundays were wholly given over to Sunday school, church, and "pass[ing] the remainder of that holy day in an orderly manner."[25] Life was undoubtedly monotonous.

Life was also drab. The frugal managers sought economy of scale in order-ing bolts of identical material for pinafores and frocks. In 1832, for example, they instructed their agent to purchase "at the North" one thousand yards of blue bombazet "of a shade which will not fade." One obvious consequence of the managers' thrift was that the girls wore an easily identifiable uniform that marked them as residents of the asylum. Signs of individuality were discour-aged; an 1860 directive instructed the matron not to allow girls to have cloth gaiters, hats, or hoops. For a time, they instituted a crackdown on colored hair ribbons, "as such things are calculated to foster a love of show & dress... which the managers consider improper." Laundresses and seamstresses exe-cuted the herculean task of maintaining the clothing of more than one hun-dred girls in decent condition. All clothing was kept in a common wardrobe room, and not until the twentieth century did the children have small lockers for their few individual possessions.[26]

While religious training and a moral education were considered essen-tial for building good character, chores were also important. A requirement that the girls work regularly alongside adult employees at cooking, scrubbing, sewing, and laundering had definite benefits. Making the children contribute to their own upkeep reduced labor costs, while practice at routine domestic chores taught girls the skills that society dictated they would need as adult women. Perhaps most important, requiring work of the girls instilled obedi-ence to authority, without which the asylum could not function.

The managers could be quite controlling. In 1859, they voted that letters to and from children at Poydras should be read by the Visiting Committee, presumably surreptitiously. Nothing in the minutes reveals what prompted adoption of this policy, nor does anything indicate that they actually carried it out. Learning that the girls were reading "improper" books and novels, they resolved to take such books away from them. Although in the Christmas sea-son the managers routinely provided a tree, dolls, toys, and candy and served a special holiday meal, they usually refused the children's requests to spend the day with friends, noting in 1871, for example, that "the outdoor influence on them has always been injurious." The effort to shield the girls from bad in-fluences extended to the residents themselves. Not uncommonly the manag-ers acted to oust girls whom they found to be in some way immoral, sending them to the House of the Good Shepherd, a nineteenth-century girls' reformatory in New Orleans operated by Catholic sisters. Of one such girl, they wrote, "She was so utterly depraved it was thought unsafe to keep her in Poydras Asylum."[27]

The goal of such interference was to "save" the girls from influences of which the managers disapproved. While, from the vantage point of the twenty-first century, such practices might seem heavy-handed, parents in middle-class homes at the time governed their own children in much the same ways, carefully and sometimes strictly regulating what they read and with whom they socialized. Like most parents of the Victorian Age, the managers approved of corporal punishment for children but cautioned the matron "to be careful to use other measures if possible." The managers fired a high-tempered cook for slapping a girl's face, and Mrs. Smith's "severity in whipping the children" led to her dismissal in 1847. When matron Mrs. Webber flailed a child with a slipper hard enough to leave "severe markings of whipping," disquieted managers judged her actions as "unduly severe." They called her to appear for questioning. After probing the circumstances of the offender's transgressions, which involved being ringleader in midnight rowdiness and rude insubordination, they chose to retain Webber in her post, but they cautioned her to avoid corporal punishment if possible and to use a paddle rather than a slipper if she felt a miscreant deserved a whipping. The unsettling episode closed with several board members earnestly talking with the girls in their schoolroom about their behavior, enjoining them to avoid a repetition of the incident.[28]

Poydras managers dispatched duties related to diet and discipline with confidence; these responsibilities fell within "the women's sphere" which the nineteenth century so strenuously insisted upon. But their crucial executive functions of planning budgets, monitoring expenses, and collecting revenue for operations inevitably led them beyond their designated domain. At no time did they experience greater financial struggles than in the half century following the Civil War; difficult though the war years had been, those that followed were harder. Those decades constitute a saga of bleak continuity, marked by tightened belts and pinched pennies. In the antebellum years, visitors to New Orleans had routinely commented about the river city's licentiousness and its wealth. In the years after the war, the frivolity and vice remained, but the city's prosperity fled. Mississippi River steamboat traffic was drastically down as passengers and freight increasingly traveled by rail; fewer and fewer bales of cotton were moved through the city's port, which seemed to be dying a slow death. A protracted economic decline ensued in the city.

The impact of hard times on the balance sheets of the Female Orphan Society was severe. In the late 1860s, the Poydras managers had collected, annually, around $25,000 in rents, income allowing them to shelter an average of ninety girls each year. They purchased provisions, clothing, stock and feed, fuel, and other necessaries; paid for repairs, salaries, insurance, and medical care; and usually finished the year with a cash balance of $2,500 to $3,500. However, for the first fifteen years after the economic downturn of 1873, Poydras Asylum income from rental properties averaged a paltry $13,700 per year. The secretary felt moved to comment on "days of gloominess and darkness, when want stares you in the face" in the summer of 1874. Average annual income for the asylum was only $14,000 in the 1890s, inching up to $17,000 in the first decade of the twentieth century. By the teens, income had nearly reached the levels of the first post–Civil War years, averaging $23,800, but annual rent did not again total the pre-panic level of $25,000 until 1915. For four long and difficult decades, then, the women of Poydras struggled to shelter and sustain their girls with severely reduced revenue. In nine of the years between 1874 and 1920, they closed the year's books with a cash balance of less than $300. And yet, paradoxically, as revenues sputtered, the old building on Magazine Street continued to serve as home to roughly the same numbers of needy children. Even with its reduced income, the Poydras Asylum sheltered an average of 87 girls in the 1870s, 90 girls in the 1880s, 113 girls in the 1890s, 91 girls in the 1900s, and 100 girls in the 1910s, while maintaining a paid staff of twelve to fifteen workers at the asylum.[29]

The women of the board managed their "loaves and fishes" miracle only by practicing the most stringent economies. Not until 1917 did they spend on provisions the amounts that they had expended forty years before. In some years, their outlay for food was only half what it had been in the 1860s while their asylum population remained more or less steady. Fortunately, their situation at the new institution on Magazine Street afforded plenty of space for cultivation of vegetables, as well as room for keeping cows and chickens. During these lean years, some questioned whether the children received adequate nourishment. An anonymous correspondent in the difficult decade of the 1870s scolded the managers for feeding the girls inadequately. Threatening embarrassing publicity unless the situation should improve quickly, the letter noted, "It is generally talked around that the children have not only very poor food but not enough of that." The writer hinted at the likelihood of "very disagreeable notice" in a city newspaper and urged better meals. It seems beyond dispute that the quality of diet at the asylum diminished considerably during the lean years.[30]

Holding the line on labor costs was another coping mechanism that brought Poydras through hard times. Not until 1915 did managers allow their workers' salaries to rise above salary levels of the immediate post–Civil War years. What passed as restraint in the eyes of the managers might well have been seen as stinginess by average workers, but the asylum's workforce was not a typical one. Many Poydras employees were residents who, upon reaching young adulthood, chose to remain in familiar surroundings and earn small wages, plus room and board, by working in laundry, kitchen, or nursery in the asylum they had known so long. Although always free to depart to establish themselves in other employment, some felt a natural attachment to the institution that had sheltered them for years. It is accurate to observe that the Poydras managers exploited this attachment to weather a difficult situation.

Part of the financial burden carried by the Poydras board concerned payments to city and state. For years, the mercurial state legislature had vacillated wildly in its approach to taxing charitable institutions, exempting some properties but not Poydras, then changing directions and extending the policy to include the Female Orphan Society as well. Board members could never know with certainty what their tax obligation might be, or whether they would even be taxed at all. In 1880, the annual report noted that a pending lawsuit for unpaid state taxes "had threatened our very existence." It took a favorable ruling by the state supreme court to remove the threat that would have "crippled if not altogether destroyed" the institution, according to the secretary. Yet, in 1903, that same court ruled that the Female Orphan Society *was* liable for taxes on its properties, a decision that necessitated the borrowing of $16,000 to pay back taxes, at a time when the society's annual income from rent was only $14,000.[31]

In such financial straits, the women deferred repairs and improvements to the home itself. Critical comments about the shabby exterior of their building pained the managers but forced them to admit that deferred maintenance had rendered it "an eyesore to ourselves and passersby." Noting that they were "continually called upon to explain" their seeming neglect, the board members, no doubt with a sigh of relief, finally saw completion of extensive "calcimining" and repairing of doors and windows in 1884, allowing the stately building to present a handsome face to the world once more. But, prudent as ever, they undertook this project only after collecting a refund of their city taxes, which they had paid under protest.[32]

Although the managers clearly preferred a "pay-as-you-go" approach, over decades of difficult budgetary circumstances the board frequently borrowed money to finance improvements on the home and on the society's stores in the business district. Correspondence with lessees makes it clear that retaining responsible tenants in commercial properties required significant outlays of money. Accordingly, the managers paid for routine maintenance, painting, and reroofing, but also for upgrades like awnings, elevators, and indoor plumbing. They went into debt in order to advance their prospects, adopting the philosophy that it takes money to make money. For example, in 1885, they borrowed fifteen thousand dollars to renovate their store on Tchoupitoulas Street, replacing a dilapidated, two-story flat-roofed building with a modern one. The completed structure, three stories tall, held five stores under one roof and was leased for $4,000 a year. At the asylum, modest expenditures upgraded the quality of life for residents and staff. In the late nineteenth century, workers installed a hot water heater for the kitchen, enlarged a dormitory, added floor coverings and new nursery furniture, and installed washers and wringers in the laundry and bathtubs in the dressing room. The welcome addition of window screens at last ended the need for cumbersome "mosquito bars" at each child's bed.

When the city of New Orleans belatedly began its long-needed modernization of water supply, sewerage, and drainage in the early twentieth century, the Poydras Asylum, like most structures, still obtained water from screened cisterns. With Sewerage and Water Board workers digging directly down Magazine Street to lay water mains, the managers in 1904 voted to connect, thus acquiring a pure and plentiful water supply at last. However, this logical step forward proved the start of a protracted process marked by many delays and a great deal of dissatisfaction with their plumbing contractor, Albert Aschaffenburg. In 1905, just when the entire house was torn up for laying the necessary pipes, the last yellow fever epidemic ever to strike the United States flared in New Orleans. The board mandated a quarantine at Poydras, and of necessity all plumbing work stopped. After a few uneasy weeks, the epidemic waned, but no sooner was the quarantine lifted than workers went on strike and deserted the thoroughly disheveled house. In all, it took three full years for plumbing to be installed properly and completely, during which time the managers were at wits' end over extensive damage done by careless workmen, their constant and disruptive presence, the lack of water pressure to the upper floors, and, as a last straw, the fetid overflowing of the buried septic tank. Board members withheld full payment to the plumber, who was not complying with his contract, hired an outside expert who recommended installing a special pump to deliver the capacity of water needed in the home, and coolly sent the bill for the necessary equipment to the hapless Mr. Aschaffenburg. Fortunately, their subsequent decision to wire the entire building for electricity in 1914 entailed no such headaches.

As the spring of 1917 approached, board members anticipated their institution's century milestone with joy, a time to celebrate one hundred years of service to indigent girls and widows. Mailing engraved invitations to a long list of dignitaries, friends, and neighbors, they ordered an immense birthday cake, supporting one hundred candles, and planned a program of prayers and oratory. Patriotic songs were also featured, appropriate because the nation had entered the First World War only one month before. After a century of service, the Poydras Asylum had earned a place in the heart of New Orleans. On this milestone, the local press saluted the institution and the women who ran it for selfless good work, noting its longevity, its quality, and its important role in the life of the city. Poydras alumnae frequently returned in adulthood to visit the old home or wrote grateful letters of reflection. Local histories rarely failed to credit the Poydras Asylum with being a landmark benevolent institution in New Orleans.

Yet nothing lasts forever. Change had been in the wings for some time and refused to wait offstage any longer. Indeed, the second century at Poydras would be nothing like the first.

8

FAREWELL TO
THE OLD POYDRAS

There was a little girl
Who had a little curl
Right in the middle of her forehead.
And when she was good she was very, very good,
But when she was bad, she was horrid.

f we should conceive the history of the Poydras Home as an orchestral symphony, robust notes of triumphalism would sound the theme for its first century; flourishes from trumpets' bright brass and brisk rhythm from tympani would indicate stout courage, steely resolution, and steady progress against all odds. But in the movement for the second century, a melancholy music plays; slower tempo and muted minor chords will serve to characterize the next fifty years at Poydras. Mournful oboes and bassoons phrase plaintive questions that seem to have no answers. In the face of abundant evidence, a half century of decline cannot be ignored, and decline undeniably plagued Poydras as it entered its second century. As the twentieth century advanced, several factors combined to force a steady reduction in the number of girls whom Poydras served. So drastic was the enrollment decline that, eventually, the Poydras board faced a situation that threatened to smother their institution's very existence. A constellation of challenging circumstances, including a troubling breakdown of discipline among the girls at Poydras, a diminishing level of involvement by the managers themselves, the rise of social work as a profession, increasing state interventions, and the severe economic hardships of the 1930s worked together to present the women of the board with a difficult choice. Daunted, but determined to carry on, in the end they faced facts, swallowed hard, and voted to change their mission. The Poydras symphony was not yet at an end.

Powerful social currents swirled far beyond the iron gates of Poydras and, inevitably, made themselves felt at the asylum. The early twentieth century is remembered as the Progressive Era, an epoch when Americans came to accept the notion that disinterested experts in the employ of government could best address troubling social problems fostered by increasing urbanization and industrialization. A corollary to this belief in professionals and government held that the day of the amateur and the volunteer, as exemplified by benevolent associations and private charitable institutions, had passed.

One aspect of progressivism involved what Americans of the Theodore Roosevelt and Woodrow Wilson eras called the "child saving" movement, dedicated to seeking a better life for all children. Zealous child welfare advocates adopted an ambitious agenda. They pressed vigorously for establishment of juvenile courts and compulsory school attendance regulations; they promoted laws to criminalize child abuse and child labor. Casting a critical eye on orphanages and condemning them as impersonal warehouses that produced maladjusted youngsters, the child-rescuers repeatedly insisted that foster homes should replace institutional care for children. Inspired by the 1909 White House Conference on Dependent Children, which had deplored the then-common practice of institutionalizing needy and neglected children, progressives also began to press successfully for "mothers' pensions," modest stipends that would allow impoverished women attempting to raise children alone to keep their families intact, in their own homes, rather than resorting to orphanages for childcare in times of financial distress. Illinois passed the first act to provide such payments in 1911, and over the next twenty years, nearly all the other states followed.[1] When President Franklin D. Roosevelt's New Deal federalized these programs under the auspices of the 1935 Social Security Act, eligible individuals began receiving federal welfare grants called Aid to Dependent Children (ADC, later AFDC, for Aid to Families with Dependent Children, and still later TANF, Temporary Assistance to Needy Families). These sweeping policy developments had significant implications for the Poydras Asylum.

Originally, the aid flowed to widowed mothers, the so-called "deserving poor." By the mid-1930s, however, other women without the support of the "normal" breadwinner were also eligible, meaning that divorced, deserted, and even never-married mothers received aid, although local governments usually acted as gatekeepers and for a time continued to sit in judgment of the so-called fitness of women who sought financial assistance. In the late 1930s, Louisiana was awarding an average of $20.18 each month to women who qualified for mothers' pensions, a niggardly sum compared to the $69.31 given in Massachusetts but more than twice as generous as the amount provided in nearby Arkansas. Slight though the amount was, it nevertheless enabled some motivated women to struggle on independently, keeping their children in the family home instead of depositing them at Poydras or other children's homes. Not coincidentally, after a spike early in the decade, Poydras enrollments declined sharply for the remainder of the 1930s. This development was almost certainly a reflection of the newly instituted ADC grants and of other New Deal programs that helped struggling families to find a modicum of security. By the presidency of Franklin Roosevelt, the Poydras Asylum was no longer the only, or even the preferred, recourse for distressed local mothers with needy children.

Even before the New Deal, various progressive reforms had affected the Poydras Asylum, private though it was. In 1909, by virtue of an amendment to the Louisiana state constitution, New Orleans established its first juvenile court, with Judge Andrew H. Wilson presiding. Wilson's court had jurisdiction over all "neglected and delinquent" children under the age of seventeen. Empowered by state law to commit such children to government-run "waifs' homes" in New Orleans, Judge Wilson also had the authority to assign these youngsters to cooperating private asylums in the city. Because the few existing state facilities were usually overcrowded, he frequently turned to the city's Catholic, Protestant, and Jewish children's homes, the Poydras Asylum among them. The Society for Prevention of Cruelty to Children, a private philanthropy, operated a children's shelter on Esplanade Avenue, and to this large, shady old house Judge Wilson sent homeless, hungry, or abused girls for temporary shelter while he attempted to arrange a permanent home for them in a local orphanage. Poydras opened its doors, as did the city's other children's homes. The judge praised the generosity and cooperation of the private institutions, noting in his first year on the bench, "We have yet to meet a refusal from any asylum or orphans' home in the city."[2]

Yet below the surface, trouble percolated at Poydras and soon boiled over. Repeated and increasingly brazen episodes of rebellious behavior, rudeness, and rule breaking among the girls crowd the pages of the Poydras managers' minutes from 1910 onward, and by the 1930s and 1940s, disharmony had become routine. Girls left the campus after dusk without permission, were "unruly," "used bad language," and showed "indifference to the rules." Ere long, some of the older girls not only refused to rise "with the rest of the family" but also refused to go to church on Sundays. In 1914, the board contacted the chief of police to request an officer to deal with gaggles of men and boys who now congregated on the street outside the gate, "using ugly language." They initially pronounced themselves pleased with the chief's response, but a year later, the nuisance continued; men and boys had begun climbing trees to look over and call down into the grounds, possibly encouraged by some on the campus. A virtual insurrection was smoldering in the once-tranquil old home.[3]

The managers responded to the crisis by embracing both traditional and modern solutions. Beyond summoning the police to deal with the male intruders, they hired a woman to teach embroidery lessons on the theory that the girls needed more to occupy their time. They called rule breakers to the boardroom and attempted to reason with them, and decided that flagrantly disobedient girls should be taken to the matron's office and "switched properly," when necessary. In a more modern spirit, they also authorized a little store in the home where girls could spend their pocket money on candies and notions, and gave permission for them to attend the neighborhood "picture show," if well chaperoned, and provided the features were "wholesome."[4]

As the years of the twentieth century passed, a frustrating dichotomy emerged involving privileges and discipline at the home. By the early 1940s, the managers were gradually extending more privileges and freedoms to the girls under their care. They allowed the superintendent to give a party for the girls every ten days during the summer and even permitted evening parties with refreshments, music, and friends invited. When girls refused to cooperate with the woman who taught sewing during the summer months, the board voted to let them go swimming instead and hired someone to do the sewing. When the girls voiced resentment at having to work at the home, the board, although convinced that daily chores built character and constituted important training for the future, for the first time entertained the idea that their workload was perhaps too heavy. The women purchased croquet, ping-pong, and badminton sets and a "victrola-radio combination" for the home. One of the managers who engaged the older girls in an informal session in which she "listened to all their desires and grievances" reported that their requests for dances, dates, and clothes were "very normal" for their ages. Making a sincere effort to address the desires of their charges, the managers converted the study hall into a recreation room, began giving allowances of spending money, and permitted the older girls to attend high school football games.[5]

The well-intentioned managers, however, sent contradictory signals to the girls at Poydras. Like most parents of this era, they came to recognize the powerful and subversive effects of peer culture. How could genteel lessons in fancy needlework compete with the beguiling temptation of adolescent boys who lounged at the corner drugstore, relaying the latest risqué jokes from the popular humor magazine *Captain Billy's WhizBang* and always ready to treat a girl for ice cream? With one hand, managers loosened restrictions and adopted certain new practices in the hope of restoring harmony and good order, but with the other, they continued to exert ill-considered attempts to maintain maximum control over all aspects of the girls' daily life. Guided by their resolute intent to shield the youngsters under their care from any influence of which they did not approve, by the 1940s they making some surprising decisions. Displeased to learn that teens who attended the St. Charles Presbyterian Church's youth fellowship were, in their view, profaning the Sabbath by playing Chinese checkers and ping-pong on Sunday evenings, they voted to withdraw permission for Poydras girls to participate. They withheld consent for them to join Girl Scout troops. They refused to allow the girls to attend a municipal picnic where they would mingle with boys and girls of other children's homes at Pontchartrain Beach. They routinely denied permission for girls to leave campus to be with friends or family on Christmas Day. By the 1950s, the board's grasp of minutiae had even expanded to include a policy regarding "stiff petticoats." In the wake of a child's tantrum of "kicking, biting and cursing" when told to remove her surplus, they solemnly decreed that one stiff petticoat would be the limit for school.

As managers tightened some controls while loosening other restrictions, discipline steadily eroded, decade after decade. A disapproving and highly inquisitive matron informed the board that Dora and Hazel "slipp[ed] out nights . . . meeting men and going to night clubs," her source being Dora's diary. Girls defiantly smoked cigarettes, skipped school, and pronounced worship services "tedious." One set of minutes after another speaks of ongoing disciplinary problems, a lack of cooperation from the older girls, and "insolence and insubordination." After stopping by the home in 1947, the board president reported the girls "most unruly" and wondered aloud "how the counselors bore it."[6]

Something had changed the atmosphere at Poydras from one of prevailing system and order, in which disciplinary infractions were rare, to an environment of near chaos. Historian Timothy Hacsi's study of orphans' homes and poor families gives us a clue. He notes that mothers' pensions for "deserving" women had the important effect of ensuring that "children whose *only* problem was their parents' poverty were now to be maintained in their parents' homes, at public expense."[7] He argues that, increasingly, the children in orphanages were primarily from homes characterized by some level of dysfunction, homes that were thus deemed ineligible for government stipends. Youngsters in children's homes often came from domestic settings plagued by violence, alcohol abuse, promiscuity, or mental illness, the "character flaws" that disqualified their parents from receiving aid. Not uncommonly, such children exhibited psychological and/or behavioral problems themselves.

Many girls mandated to Poydras by Judge Wilson and his successors over the years really were more troubled and thus more difficult than the usual population of the home, and certainly they contributed to the change in the tone of operations there. However, it seems far too Manichean to cite the entry of girls sent by the juvenile court as the sole factor contributing to the troubles. Girls from troubled backgrounds were not the only youngsters being admitted. Furthermore, just at a time when intelligent supervision had a greater-than-ever role to play at the asylum, board minutes show that Poydras managers had drifted into a pattern of inconsistent engagement. Undeniably, they were spending less time at the home than ever before. Adopting a stance that would have stunned their tirelessly energetic predecessors, they often allowed an ill-qualified superintendent to have the final say in important policy matters, noting with detachment that "she is living on the place and would know better as to the advisability than the Managers." This practice later resulted in steady complaints, unparalleled in asylum history, alleging that the loosely supervised, underpaid staff slapped, spanked, and severely whipped the children. At one point in the 1930s, the board members' detachment was such that they were shocked to learn, belatedly, that the home's superintendent regularly stayed out late at night with a male companion and compensated by sleeping late in the mornings; they also heard charges that the man had inappropriately fondled the girls. By the 1950s, a growing lack of personal interest led to a decision that the once-active visiting committee would no longer come to the home at all unless specifically summoned by the superintendent. Though less of a presence at the home and less involved in setting important policies such as appropriate measures of punishment, the managers paradoxically embroiled themselves in trivial matters, spending valuable minutes on a discussion about authorizing purchase of a muzzle after the mule had bitten the gardener, and pausing to vote on whether Juanita might receive a raincoat for Christmas.[8]

In the nineteenth century, when there were no term limits, zealous managers had served on the Poydras board for decades. Finding in the work a welcome outlet for their executive abilities, the most active and influential women spent massive amounts of time and energy dealing with the home and its occupants; they were talented, enthusiastic, and committed women. Three stalwarts—Phoebe Laidlaw, Clemence Toby, and Mary Luzenberg—had combined to labor for Poydras for over 150 years before their deaths in 1878, 1879, and 1881, respectively. Beyond dispute, they truly *knew* the asylum, root, branch, and in all seasons. But times had changed by the twentieth century, when, for example, in the dark and difficult year of 1938, two managers and the president abruptly resigned from the board without completing even one term, abandoning the ship in stormy seas. Worried remaining members undertook a heartfelt discussion about how to recruit properly motivated replacements for those dispirited managers who fell by the wayside. Echoing the tone of crisis, the author of the 1938 annual report looked to the past and pointedly saluted "good and true women who met in session, in this room, at this table, in years gone by, [who] gave of their time, toil and prayers, their labor only ceasing with the close of their long and useful lives." She closed by imploring the current crop to "emulate these lovable characters and . . . carry on."[9]

Not only were twentieth-century managers less involved in operation of the home itself, they had also surrendered financial decisions almost totally.

John B. Ferguson, husband of treasurer Phoebe Raymond Ferguson and an officer of Whitney Bank, seems to have been given *carte blanche* in handling rentals, taxes, bills, and investments. Getting recommendations from male advisers had long been standard practice among the women, but the boards of the 1920s and 1930s virtually abdicated fiduciary responsibility. It was Ferguson, for example, who came before the board and acquainted the women with the dire situation regarding their outstanding bills in 1935, a situation that unaccountably took them quite by surprise. It was Ferguson who urged the managers to borrow to cover their debts until he could collect their rents and Ferguson alone who held permission to open a safe deposit box held for the managers at Whitney Bank. It was Ferguson who contacted the president of the city's board of assessors to request a reduction in assessments of Poydras rental properties. And it was Ferguson who floated a plan for furnishing and fitting out the old Campbell mansion as an apartment house in the hope of generating income. Exactly how and why this abdication of responsibility occurred is not clear, but it represents a great departure from the hands-on approach followed during the nineteenth century. In those years, the managers had, at intervals, readily sought the counsel of male advisers, but they never appeared less than conversant with the affairs of the asylum they managed, in deed as well as in name.[10]

When John Ferguson died, on the eve of World War II, the managers engaged the Trust Department of Whitney Bank to manage their stocks and bonds in exchange for 5 percent of all revenue. They negotiated with Leo Fellmann's real estate company to manage their real estate holdings and insurance arrangements, at a fee of 6 percent of gross rentals. They relied more than ever on the advisory committee, which at that point included Ashton Phelps, Leeds Eustis, and Watts K. Leverich.

Perhaps much of the board's dependence had roots in the 1930s, the venerable institution's darkest decade, when troubles crashed over Poydras in waves. Revenues of course declined. Some businesses that leased Poydras properties ceased paying rent altogether and ultimately defaulted (Capitol City Auto Company and the Chalmette Hotel, for example), while others managed to make payment only by demanding and receiving sizable rent reductions (Toye Brothers Yellow Cab Company). When Canal Bank & Trust failed, Poydras deposits went down with it. Repeatedly the managers accepted mere cents on the dollar when bonds matured, as the issuers lacked funds to pay in full; often issuers notified the women that they would offer only greatly reduced rates of interest.

Amidst severe challenges, the managers retrenched with vigor, slashing all staff salaries by 10 percent and instructing the matron to reduce the portions of meat and milk being served to children. Other than salmon croquets on Fridays and stewed chicken on Sundays, meat disappeared altogether from the menus, replaced by a heavy reliance on grits, oatmeal, and macaroni and cheese. When a powerful storm rattled the asylum and caused a cataract of leaks in the roof, the managers merely ordered pots and pans placed strategically and repaired only what was absolutely necessary; their treasury dictated that the rest must wait. When the heating system ceased to work properly, they deferred repairs and urged everyone to bundle up. In 1935 they paid city and state property taxes only by holding back on paying some of their bills and resorting to a loan. Times were sufficiently rocky that the managers even countenanced violating a longstanding principle and selling off a portion of their original Julien Poydras inheritance. However, the beleaguered board's flickering hope that the U.S. government would purchase Poydras property at Julia and Carondelet Streets as the site for a new federal building came to nothing.

Even as Poydras revenues stagnated, relentless Depression conditions increased the need for shelter for disadvantaged girls. Distressing circumstances among applicants, such as the frightened little girl sharing a bed with her impoverished and epileptic mother who was experiencing increasingly violent fits at night, or the full orphan living a tenuous existence with a nearly destitute family of nine children, led the women to order additional beds for the dormitories. With the wolf at the door, they overcame their ingrained suspicion of the government sufficiently to apply for and begin receiving commodities from the Federal Emergency Relief Administration. The government's largesse included hundreds of pounds of rice, sugar, canned meats, and flour, as well as great quantities of onions, grapefruits, and prunes. However, it was outright deception that opened the way for such generous distribution of foodstuffs; the asylum supervisor, Mrs. Riche, gave undeniably false information in the home's application for commodity distribution from the Works Progress Administration (WPA). Riche signed a sworn statement that the home cared for 135 girls, but just one month later, an in-house roster showed only 82 children in residence. There is no evidence that the managers were party to this deception, but there is no evidence that they were not. In previous years, an alert and thoroughly engaged board would have detected such falsehoods in the ordinary exercise of their management. That Mrs. Riche felt emboldened to resort to such easily provable dishonesty either indicates her confidence that she was but loosely supervised or shows that the managers approved her deception.

The asylum gratefully received hundreds of well-made robes, towels, and quilts from the sewing rooms of the WPA, enjoyed the tutoring contributions of Sophie Newcomb College students who were paid by the National Youth Administration, and sent girls to WPA-funded piano lessons. Mayor Robert Maestri, a warm friend to the asylum, indicated his continuing interest in the institution by annually inviting a Poydras girl to join him in reviewing the Rex parade each year on Carnival Day and to have the honor of presenting a key to the city to the king. Maestri's appropriation of WPA funds for asylum repairs and his periodic visits to the children thrilled the managers. Yet in 1934, they voted to reject the monthly stipend of thirty dollars customarily paid to them by the city, because they objected to revealing details about their institution's finances, admissions, and discharges to New Orleans's newly established Department of Public Welfare.

Indeed, the managers had long looked with distrust upon all the outside entities that had attempted to gain information pertaining to the asylum's financial position and operating procedures. In this posture, they were not at all unusual. The authors of a 1910 "Report on Benevolent Institutions," compiled by the U.S. Census Bureau, had confessed the impossibility of obtaining the desired data from privately operated institutions, many of whose directors "objected to making public their private finances."[11] Progressives persisted in their efforts to monitor private institutions in the name of public interest, but Poydras parried all thrusts from the outside and declined to open ledgers or share policies with inquisitive interlopers. Although the managers heard increasingly from the Board of Charities and Corrections, the Council of Social Agencies, the Louisiana Department of Public Welfare, the Child Welfare Department of New Orleans, the Family Services Society, the State Board of Health, and the state fire marshal, they managed to dodge, divert, or delay requests for policy changes and statistical information. A 1904 law gave the Board of

Charities and Corrections authority to visit all private charitable institutions, but power to supervise only state-run facilities. When Dr. Maud Loeber, the inspector from the Board of Prisons and Asylums in New Orleans, visited Poydras, she complimented the appearance of the girls, but whether she and other social workers and government functionaries liked what they found there or not, the managers steadfastly refused to reveal details of their budgets and policies. When the Council on Social Agencies inquired about upkeep costs and admission requirements at Poydras in early 1941, the board of managers voted to "answer the letter in a polite but brief way," but to provide no information. Their private sources of revenue allowed them to spurn the Community Chest, which required full disclosures from entities applying for funds. The Poydras board clearly felt no need for more supervision or oversight.[12]

As the century progressed, Poydras managers were discovering a new breed of "intruder," the professional social worker. Social work, a classic example of the progressive spirit at work, aimed to empower its practitioners to improve the quality of life for individuals and groups. The university-trained social worker gathered copious data about clients in need of help, devised and implemented action plans, and then monitored and evaluated the situation. In New Orleans, Tulane University offered courses in social work as early as 1914 and, with a grant from the Rockefeller Foundation, expanded its program and gained national accreditation in 1927. The influential and capable New Orleanian Elizabeth Wisner, who earned her Ph.D. at the University of Chicago, took the helm of Tulane's School of Social Work in the 1930s. Wisner shaped the school into a prestigious institution and began producing a corps of ambitious, motivated social workers, many of whom found work in the city. From them came a barrage of invitations and requests to Poydras, urging the managers and staff to attend workshops and seminars, to adopt social worker–designated "best practices" at their institution, and to divulge data so that the asylum could be represented in annuals and statistical summaries then being regularly compiled. They encouraged managers to bone up on child welfare theories, to keep case histories in a methodical manner, to regularize admission and withdrawal procedures, and to allow graduate students in social work to conduct studies at the Poydras Home.

The managers were soon enmeshed in a paradox. They clearly preferred to keep their institutional information private. But though they had long dis-

trusted professional children's advocates, they dealt increasingly with a population of girls whose emotional and behavioral problems outstripped the
abilities of well-meaning volunteers and underpaid staff to help them. Gradually, the managers began to seek professional help for their charges. For example, they requested advice and sometimes services from the professionals
at the Child Guidance Center, the Children's Bureau, the Child Conservation
League, the Child Welfare Department, and Tulane's School of Social Work.
They turned to public agencies to make psychiatric evaluations of children;
they approached the clinic at Touro Hospital for help with the mounting
problem of bed wetters; they relied on social workers for advice about admissions. Almost without realizing it, the managers leaned more and more
heavily on outside agencies and individuals. Dependence on the expertise of
others was ultimately a solvent that eroded the managers' trust in their own
instincts regarding the Poydras Asylum. As they outsourced more and more
functions, the distance grew between women of the board and the institution
they served.

Not entirely without reason, midcentury managers began to question the
wisdom of continuing to operate Phoebe Hunter's cherished female orphan
asylum at all. As early as 1941, Poydras representatives had heard a consultant on foster care for the state of Louisiana speak frankly about trends in
child welfare. She emphasized to her audience that the time was coming when
children's homes would need to redefine their purpose. They listened as she
methodically built her case, deploying solid evidence. Falling mortality rates
and greater longevity meant that the full orphan was rare indeed. Governmen-
tal financial aid now ensured that economic insecurity alone could not force
struggling parents to deposit their children at facilities like Poydras. Thanks to
universally accepted progressive ideas, a fairly adequate system of foster care
sheltered many children who could not live with neglectful or abusive birth
families deemed unfit to care for them. The once-radical notion, born in the
progressive era, that children should be cared for in homes of their own, had
taken root; a new system now provided alternatives to institutional congregate
care for needy and neglected girls.

Statistics clearly show the impact of these trends. While the population of
the United States grew robustly, the number of children in institutional care
declined from a high of 144,000 in the mid-1930s to only 95,000 in 1951. Poy-

dras reflected the national trend. Enrollment plummeted from a Depression-era high of 91 to an average of only 35 in the 1940s and 1950s. In the main, the girls at the Poydras Asylum were not forced there by dire poverty, and there were few whole or half orphans. Instead, many Poydras girls were youngsters whose home life was deemed unstable, whose behavioral, emotional, and personality problems made them unable to secure assignment to a foster home, or whose surviving parent would not permit such assignment.

Records show that, in 1937, for example, the Poydras population of seventy girls included only ten full orphans and fifteen half orphans; the other forty-five girls had two living parents. Some terse notations made by the matron indicate the painful conditions of many of their lives: "Location of mother unknown; father in insane hospital in Texas"; "mother in Florida, ill and unemployed; father in South America. Does not keep in touch with girls"; "Placed by Children's Burea [sic]. Mother deserted children and father contributes nothing"; "Mother in State Hospital; Father visits occasionally; sometimes gives Valerie a few nickels"; "No one visits her. Family scattered."[13]

Many, though not all, Poydras girls in these decades were troubled and unreachable, or disruptive and rebellious, in need of special social and psychiatric services. But the idea of becoming a residential care facility (or "group home," as the new jargon put it), dispensing therapy for troubled girls and adolescents, held little appeal for the heirs of the nineteenth-century founders. Wearied by intractable problems that left them feeling inadequate, and confronting the stark reality of falling enrollments, the women of the Poydras board began to tiptoe toward a once-unthinkable possibility.

Developments of the 1940s and 1950s gave them a hearty shove toward a new mission. The venerable old building on Magazine Street was deteriorating fast as it approached its hundredth birthday in 1957. Termites had wreaked silent but serious havoc. Ceilings were collapsing. Massive cast-iron decorations and a heavy cement cornice over the Corinthian columns threatened to fall. Dispirited managers scrutinized their structure and wondered whether to repair, replace, or sell. Tentatively, they began to learn more about the cottage system, small units where eight or ten children lived with a housemother in modern, independent, homelike residences scattered about a campus. They visited other children's homes to note the number and duties of staff there. Clearly, they were casting about, trying to find a way forward. In

1950, however, the board came within one vote of passing a motion to sell their entire property to New Orleans activist Elizabeth Miller Robin for her dream of building a hospital for crippled children. Later that year, representatives of the city's Ochsner Clinic approached the managers about their wish to purchase the entire Poydras Asylum site for the new hospital they were planning, but the women replied that the property was not for sale and explained that they were "considering plans for a home for the aged."[14]

This comment stands as the first mention of eldercare at Poydras. Existing records do not clarify just how the managers happened to contemplate converting their institution to a home for the elderly. In fact, for several years in the 1950s, the board remained divided about a course of action, agreeing only that the status quo was untenable. Because of uncertainty, they delayed all but the most routine repairs on the home. Consultation with their advisory committee and with architects convinced them initially that their old building was fundamentally sound and eminently worth saving, although in need of extensive and costly repairs, and further, that the cost of building new, for any endeavor, would be prohibitively expensive.

As the beleaguered board hesitated over which path to take, news came that state licensing of residential childcare facilities would be required for all institutions at the end of 1957. Proving burdensome in the extreme, this mandate forced the hand of the managers at Poydras, who now confronted a perfect storm of difficulties in meeting various standards. Regulations from the state fire marshal presented a tremendous obstacle. Steep staircases, impossible to negotiate with speed, led down from the third-floor dormitory, where metal grillwork, intended to deter nighttime truancy among the girls, covered the windows. The children lived in a veritable firetrap. Bringing the old home up to standards would involve moving all girls off the third floor, enclosing the open staircases, installing expensive sprinkler systems throughout, and instituting a system of regular fire drills.

Meanwhile, turmoil flared among the underpaid staff members at the home, as they were proving contentious and uncooperative in this time of trouble. Turnover was again a problem. Consultants stated flatly that the managers should hire better-educated workers of higher caliber and thereby eliminate the twin problems of professionalism and retention. Only better pay would accomplish these goals, however, and it was not forthcoming. The women of the board made overtures to various religious leaders, all male, asking if they would serve as the home's superintendent; all declined. A manager who visited the home during this season found conditions "deplorable" and reported, "The girls have no discipline, there is utter confusion at mealtime, the staff members and domestics are discontented and the superintendent is not available at any time." Just at this juncture, teachers at the public school suspended several Poydras girls for continued misbehavior, and to cap the climax, dark rumors began to circulate in the community alleging mistreatment and neglect of the children. The frustrated board president, Marion Lyons, concluded her annual report for 1956 by observing wearily, "I am sure you agree that neither the making nor the spending of the money of Mr. Poydras … caused … any more worry than it has each one of us, but we pray for guidance and courage to carry on."[15]

Although facing a policy decision of momentous proportions, one that required careful study, the managers nevertheless could not abandon their old habit of micromanaging affairs at the home. Board minutes show them instructing the staff to let the younger children watch the television shows *Ding Dong School* and *Big Top* and voting to deny privileges to Bobbie, whose teachers reported that she had "a flip attitude and lack of study." They even listened attentively as the home administration committee chair explained earnestly why she recommended spraying for roaches but not fogging for mosquitoes at the institution. Somehow, amid this welter of self-imposed and energy-depleting details, they groped their way toward a crucial policy choice.[16]

In the mid-1950s, the managers had begun enrolling a few of the older girls at either the Holmes Junior College High School or the French Camp Academy, both in rural Mississippi.[17] Sending adolescents away to boarding school removed disruptive influences from Poydras, and the board members had been more than willing to assume costs of tuition and board in their futile quest for tranquility. Neither this solution nor any other had proved adequate to their storm of problems, however.

Shortly before Thanksgiving, 1957, parents of the few girls still under the care of Poydras received, by registered mail, a startling letter. The board of managers had at last reached a decision about the future. The brief letter stated that the Poydras Home (which had only recently begun styling itself as "Home" rather than "Asylum," in acquiescence to demands from the girls and recommendations from social agencies)[18] would soon close in order to be converted to a home for elderly ladies. Citing as justification the duplication of services with existing children's homes and a belief that the need for eldercare was greater than that for residential care for children, the unexpected letter gave surprised adults a mere one month's notice that their children would be permanently dismissed to parental custody after the home's annual Christmas party. Several girls expressed anger at the abrupt dismissal. The efficient wardrobe committee nonetheless packed up the girls' few belongings and, at parting, gave them all that remained of the institution's toys and bicycles.

And thus, with the release of the twelve surprised girls to their presumably stunned parents, only five nights before Christmas, 1957, 140 distinguished years of the Female Orphan Society's history came to a peremptory close.[19]

9

AND WELCOME TO THE NEW!

We never know how high we are
Till we are called to rise;
And then, if we are true to plan,
Our statures touch the skies.

Q. How do you eat an elephant?
A. One bite at a time.

In the late 1950s, the fifteen unpaid women on the Poydras board of managers confronted their own particular elephant in the form of the Poydras Home's future. After dispiriting years of presiding over decline as their venerable institution drifted on a sea of chaos, after agonizing discussions around the big mahogany table in the boardroom, they had at last made a firm determination to shift from serving the young to helping the elderly.

Vexing headaches soon replaced the relief they felt at ending their troubled effort to continue serving girls. New issues plagued the well-intentioned managers. Of immediate importance was the question of how the physical structure should be amended to care for the elderly. In 1958, with the building standing empty for the first time in one hundred years, the managers summoned demolition experts for an evaluation. Could the old three-story home be whittled down to only one floor, thus keeping the architectural integrity of the original structure while eliminating the costly fire safety renovations now required for a three-story building? After careful inspection, the initial consultants advised against removing the top two floors; the expense would be prohibitive, they declared. Subsequent conversations with their architect convinced the board that the most economical and practical course was demolition. Accordingly, and somewhat surprisingly, given their oft-stated respect for history and continuity, the women voted without dissent to demolish the old Poydras Asylum, first occupied in 1857, creation of Lewis Reynolds and home to hundreds of girls across an entire century. They determined to replace it with a completely new structure of midcentury modern design.

Thankfully, two months later came a turning point. Olin J. Farnsworth, chairman of R. P. Farnsworth & Co., the largest contracting and construction firm in Louisiana, appeared before the board to make an impassioned plea to save the original orphanage. He and his chief engineer had inspected the old building carefully; their tour had convinced them of the feasibility of removing the top two floors and renovating the ground floor for use by elderly residents, and, Farnsworth added with emphasis, "*Think what you would have.*" The knowledge that they were "custodians of a fine example of the building art" warred strenuously with "the urge to be practical and economical," as the president's annual report candidly admitted. After Farnsworth's timely and persuasive intervention, however, the women rescinded their vote to demolish and opted instead for reduction to one story, coupled with renovation of the existing historic structure. Preservation had carried the day.[1]

Dismantling and removal of the top two floors took place in 1959. However, the managers' chosen architect, Earl Mathes of the well-known firm Favrot Reed Mathes & Bergman, hesitated. Guided by their dictum to spend as little as possible, Mathes had already drawn plans for a modern building to replace the Lewis Reynolds structure and seemed reluctant to change course. He was particularly disinclined to have the women turn for consultation, as they proposed, to Samuel Wilson, Jr., architect and dean of historic preservationists in the city. Offering to sketch other options, more in keeping with the existing architecture, Mathes urged against bringing Wilson into the process. Still enamored of his own original design, he continued to press the Poydras board to accept his less costly and more modern approach. As the women worked to reach an important decision about the roof, which would strongly influence the look of the entire edifice, board president Marion Lyons asked Mathes if they should at least inform the Louisiana Landmarks Society of their plans. "I do not think it advisable," he responded. Finally, the roofing contractor they had hired told the managers emphatically that he believed "it was worth every nickel of the cost to make something of our fine building ... [and] spend the additional money [to add a more steeply pitched roof]." The vacillating board of managers swung back to the preservationist viewpoint and voted in the end to accept the expensive, more historically appropriate roof. The lovely structure of today thus came within a very near miss of looking a great deal like a nondescript suburban motel. In the end, to placate Mathes, the managers did not consult the eminent Wilson but settled for writing flattering letters to him and to Martha Gilmore Robinson, the Landmarks Society's first president, stressing that the managers understood their "responsibility as custodians of a 'landmark.'" Both Wilson and Robinson received invitations to the open house for the newly remodeled Poydras Home, and both attended. This initial cordiality would not immunize the Poydras board from the wrath of preservationists a few years later, however.[2]

Important questions awaited answers as construction proceeded. How should the new facility be equipped? Initially, the managers planned to fit out the existing structure to accommodate perhaps a dozen elderly women residents, with the intent to grow as soon as possible. The expansion they envisioned would be a modern wing for bedroom units, allowing them to avoid cannibalizing the original structure. Keeping intact most of the large rooms, with their sixteen-foot ceilings, mammoth marble fireplaces, and beautiful mill- and plasterwork, retained the old building's antebellum graciousness. The long-range plan called for the original structure to house parlors, dining rooms, offices, and an infirmary. To ready the one-time orphanage for its debut as a retirement facility, managers turned out in numbers to work at the home, and the *Times-Picayune* approvingly reported their performance of "domestic chores … such as supervising gardening, rearranging furniture, decorating, studying the effect of candlesticks on pianos and centerpieces on tables," fondly noting their "cheerfulness and enthusiasm." But the newspaper's account pastoralized the women's contributions. In fact, quite beyond merely supervising the exertions of others, they gave hard physical labor, working, steadily, at sanding and painting old iron bedsteads from the attic and varnishing cast-off bedside tables from the Roosevelt Hotel. The board president explained their frugality by noting that "our prime function is service, not things."[3]

Who should be allowed to reside at the Poydras Home? Board members chose to review all applications for admission themselves, scrutinizing every aspect of a prospective resident's personality, health, and financial status, screening rigorously. Operating a wholly private facility, they initially stipulated that all residents be ambulatory, able to care for themselves personally, and in acceptable physical condition as determined by a mandatory examination by Dr. John Phillips, their medical director. A handicap of "mental illness," by which the managers meant any sort of dementia, was a disqualifying factor. They rejected other applicants for morbid obesity, advanced age and debility, and, more ominously, "for numerous reasons discovered in the inquiry." A probationary period of three months allowed the managers to dismiss a resident if they felt she was not in fact a good match for life at Poydras. The managers justified ousting probationary residents by noting "personality problems . . . does not integrate well into a home atmosphere," "doesn't adjust to institutional living," and "needs too much personal attention." Basing monthly fees on a sliding scale, tied to a resident's ability to pay, they made financial assistance available to those who had demonstrable need. They turned no one away because of lack of financial resources; indeed, they subsidized nearly every resident in the early years. They nevertheless rejected many applicants. In 1962, for example, of thirty-nine who applied, only eight gained admission. In their quest to select a certain type of resident, the managers employed chiefly unstated although seemingly understood criteria. One condition was written quite specifically into their constitution, however: "only white Protestant women" would find a home at Poydras.[4]

By spring of 1960, the managers had accepted the first four residents for the new Poydras Home for Elderly Ladies, and within a few months, the home's census stood at seventeen, housed in rather spartan shared quarters, chiefly double rooms and a four-bed ward, with only two single rooms available in that first year. Yet serving so few residents entailed a relatively high per capita cost of operation. Uncertain about demand for the service they offered and equally uncertain about their capacity to manage the new undertaking of geriatric care, the managers by intent had started slowly. Eighteen months of reasonable success dissolved their doubts, however, and in autumn 1961, they confidently broke ground for new space to accommodate twenty more women. In a year's time, they occupied this "1960s Wing," more than doubling the home's capacity. A longtime board member reverently quoted Psalm 127 at the time of its dedication: "Except the Lord build the house, they labor in vain who build it." Noting that the old order of the original asylum for helpless girls had given way to the new Poydras Home for the elderly, she added, "Some things never change; among them the need of helping those who cannot meet their own needs."[5]

Several recurring issues preoccupied the managers as they steered the Poydras Home in its new mission. First of all, inadequate salaries and lack of professional personnel hampered the success of the institution in its early years. When the asylum housed girls, the Poydras board had routinely relied on nonprofessionals in supervisory positions, often hiring genteel widows who needed work and who possessed more or less adequate knowledge of housekeeping, nutrition, and record keeping. In the last chaotic years of the asylum's existence, many outsiders had urged the managers to hire, and to compensate properly, a competent professional administrator, but to no avail.

The pattern of eschewing professional staff continued when the home opened to serve the elderly. Indeed, the Poydras Home operated for two full decades before the managers opted to hire a licensed superintendent who had actually passed the examinations administered by the state of Louisiana for nursing home administrators.[6] Until that time, they left the day-to-day functioning of Poydras in the hands of a series of nurses, women who individually had some sterling qualities—such as a warm personality, or a special knowledge of health issues among the elderly, or even an ability to play the piano to entertain the residents—but who lacked the skill sets needed in the crucial position of administrator. The managers continued to insist on authority over any but the slightest expenditures, making all large purchases for the home themselves, investing the time to compare prices before buying an icemaker or a lawnmower, for example, and hiring the washing machine repairman personally. At the same time, an ingrained reluctance to pay wages that compared favorably with those offered at other homes for the elderly resulted in tremendous staff turnover. Not only was pay for cooks and nurses' aides decidedly low, but benefits were at first nonexistent.

A second recurring theme for Poydras managers concerned their profound distrust of the federal government. The Poydras Home's status as a fully private facility allowed the board of managers great autonomy in setting policies, and they intended to keep it. For decades, they had deflected inquiries from state and local agencies when the home sheltered youngsters, and their wariness continued. In 1965 the board president lamented "harassments by man and by nature," which she identified bluntly as "the passing of the Civil Rights Act . . . and the visitation of Hurricane Betsy." A query from the U.S. Department of Health, Education, and Welfare (HEW) asking if the institution intended to comply with the recently adopted Civil Rights Act of 1964 prompted a flurry of questions from the managers to Poydras attorneys and the advisory board, after which the managers voted to continue admitting only white Protestant women.[7] This decision for noncompliance meant that they forfeited state financial assistance to Poydras residents who were deemed "needy." Monthly government checks had to this point helped some residents pay their fees at the home. Deprived of this revenue because of the admissions policy, the managers chose to increase the subsidies they provided for women in need, whose ability to pay for care now fell far short of the monthly amount being spent on them. The managers much preferred extra expense to federal oversight, a viewpoint confirmed by outside consultant Dr. Robert Elsasser of Tulane University's business school, who in 1969 advised them to continue their noncompliance with the Civil Rights Act because of what he termed "the multitude of constricting conditions imposed by the Federal government."[8]

Through the 1960s, the home consistently spent more money than it took in. Between 1961 and 1969, income increased about 33 percent while food costs doubled and expenditures for salaries quadrupled. In their worry over the facility's financial situation, and seeking to end a hemorrhage of funds, the managers inadvertently blundered into a swarm of criticism that stung them painfully. Weary of the effort required to keep their struggling apartment house at St. Charles and Julia Streets in the black, convinced that it would never turn a steady profit, they announced plans to raze the structure. Known to the public as the Campbell Mansion, the grand old structure represented only a money pit to the managers. However, preservationists saw it quite differently. General Benjamin Butler had commandeered this gracious antebellum home for use as his residence during the Union occupation of New Orleans; it was rightly considered a property of notable historic and architectural importance. The fledgling preservationist movement, in the form of the Louisiana Landmarks Society, raised an outcry, calling on the board of managers to rescind their decision or to allow them extra time to raise money to purchase the mansion themselves. Remarking crisply that their mission was to "preserve old lives, not old buildings," the unmoved managers bid the wrecking ball do its work. When the dust had settled, the dark utilitarian asphalt of a parking lot had replaced a beautiful historic building. The ugly flat surface shimmered in the midday heat, a silent affront to all local preservationists, who freely and repeatedly expressed their outrage to Poydras managers in person and in the public press.[9]

While reeling from negative publicity, the board continued to grapple with a situation in which disbursements at the Poydras Home exceeded income by an alarming margin. In 1968 residents paid a total of $47,000 while expenses ran to $117,000. If allowed to continue, such a situation would threaten the very existence of the Poydras enterprise. The costs of operating a small home were disproportionately great, and not surprisingly, troubled conversations about revenue occupied the managers at every meeting. Had they bitten off more than they could chew in attempting to operate a home for the elderly? After 150 years of continuous operation in New Orleans, through hurricanes and epidemics, bank panics and Federal occupation, would the iconic Poydras Home cease to exist because *they* had failed, when all their predecessors on the board had managed to succeed? The Poydras managers doggedly focused on ways to increase the income from their real estate holdings; somehow, they must stanch the red ink on their ledger books. Then, at last, after a dreary half century of downward spiral and troubles in flocks, their luck changed. The sun came out. They found a way.

Thanks to a chain of related events, New Orleans was at this time poised for a boom, the epicenter of which would be the so-called "Poydras Corridor." The timing could not have been more fortuitous. When the decade of the 1960s opened, Poydras Street, just four blocks upriver from the city's commercial district on and near Canal Street, squatted over what had once been a fetid canal; lined with ramshackle buildings, it was an undistinguished, narrow roadway that truckers avoided. A few years and four million dollars later, purposeful demolition and construction had nearly doubled the roadway's width. Completed in the summer of 1966, the revamped Poydras Street, a nicely landscaped, 134-foot-wide boulevard featuring six lanes and a 22-foot neutral ground, became the attractive approach to the city's new Trade Mart Complex and the Rivergate Convention Center, then rising on the river and nearing completion. Shortly, One Shell Square, at a soaring fifty-one stories the tallest building in Louisiana, claimed its address at 701 Poydras. At the other end of the street, pile drivers pounded and concrete mixers rumbled to erect the state's pride, the Louisiana Superdome, the building of which had been a caveat of local businessman Dave Dixon's brash deal to win a National Football League franchise for New Orleans. When the Saints brought professional football to the Crescent City, big hotels followed, and Poydras Street was home to a Hyatt by 1976 and a Hilton by 1980. The fifteen blocks of Poydras between the river and the Dome soon sprouted ranks of high-rise office towers, gleaming projectiles of glass and granite fit to house the entrepreneurs of a sudden oil boom that splashed prosperity into the region in the 1970s. In 1982, a World's Fair would begin to rise in New Orleans on an eighty-two-acre site located in this vicinity. Property on Poydras Street was hot. And the women of the Poydras Home's board of managers held some prime pieces.[10]

Only months before the widening project on Poydras Street reached completion, New Orleans developer Joseph Canizaro floated an offer of $80,000 to the women. He wanted to lease their property at 300 Poydras, then home to the Pelican Banana Company, and build one of the first skyscrapers on the refurbished thoroughfare. They demurred. His next offer of $100,000, made only one month later, gave them a shrewd idea that, as their minutes put it, "we have not yet seen the top of real estate prices there."[11] They were content to sit tight, and, ultimately, Canizaro paid $300,000 to lease the site where he erected the Lykes Building. Rising prices for real estate on Poydras Street spilled over to adjacent areas, including nearby Julia and Carondelet Streets. In the coming years, Poydras managers negotiated lease renewals with tenants of Poydras properties on those streets at handsomely increased rates. In 1982 alone, gross income from all Poydras real estate holdings skyrocketed by a stunning 87 percent.

But there was more good luck to come. Just as revenue began to gush from land that Julien Poydras had left to the Female Orphan Society some 150 years before, the women fielded a flurry of inquiries from interested parties about their unused square of ground situated adjacent to the Poydras Home itself. Local real estate titans Latter & Blum and Waguespack-Pratt, and developers Robert Walmsley and Ronald Brignac, all expressed interest in building housing on the Uptown site at Jefferson and Laurel Streets. However, it was a proposal from the New Orleans Lawn Tennis Club that most piqued the interest of the board. With plans to build a clubhouse, a pool, and twelve tennis courts, the well-heeled NOLTC impressed the managers as likely to be a good neighbor who would create neither noise nor litter, and in 1972, the parties signed a lease, giving Poydras just under $25,000 annually for the first ten years, with options for renewal for additional periods up to eighty-nine years, at an amount to be adjusted every ten years by appraisal.

Another windfall materialized in 1973. The well-regarded Fink Home, also known as the Delachaise Home, announced plans for closure. Built by a wealthy importer just after the Civil War, this elegant Italianate house on Camp Street had become the Fink Home when the city of New Orleans purchased it with funds left by realtor John David Fink. In accord with Fink's will, the city operated it as an asylum for Protestant widows. When, after nearly a century, the home found it too costly to comply with various code regulations from fire and health departments, its board voted to give all of the Fink assets to the Poydras Home, provided only that some future construction on the Poydras campus be named to honor their patron. Thus, Poydras realized another gain, over $200,000 in securities and the Fink property itself, which they sold in 1975 for $310,000. Also in 1975, the city of New Orleans purchased a small slice of Poydras-owned property on Poydras Street, planning to incorporate it with other land parcels to create the flamboyant Piazza d'Italia, and the board of managers pocketed another $375,000.

Thus, almost as if by divine intervention, the women of Poydras saw their financial situation transformed in a surprisingly brief period. The oil boom bathed New Orleans in prosperity; an economic takeoff ensued in the 1960s and 1970s. The development of the Poydras Corridor caused real estate prices in that vicinity to skyrocket. Eager developers leased what had long ago been a part of Julien Poydras's plantation, and the managers wisely renegotiated existing leases at higher rates. Serendipity played a role as well; the tennis club deal was lucrative, and the Fink assets dropped into their laps as if from heaven. Even an offer they wanted to refuse had a silver lining. Loath to sell one square foot of the original legacy from benefactor Poydras, committed as always to their longstanding policy of leasing instead, the women learned that the city, bent on creating the Piazza d'Italia as a public square to honor New Orleanians of Italian descent, had already acquired every parcel of land that it needed, with the exception of their Poydras lot, and was threatening expropriation if they balked at selling. Reluctantly, they sold, and realized a cool $375,000. From a host of sources, money rolled in. Their only dilemma was what to do with it. Not for the first time, the managers nodded knowingly to each other and murmured their mantra, "Poydras prayers are always answered."

Finding themselves thus thoroughly liberated from economic worries after a long and vexing season of money troubles, the managers did not rest on their oars. Board president Charlotte Carter Smith in 1972 stated ambitiously, "It is really criminal to spend the amount of money we spend on caring for 26 residents. With just a little expenditure and more competent management, I feel like we could care for twice as many ladies."[12] The waiting list for the Poydras Home had tripled in only three years. Women of the board felt troubled to know that they were rejecting many applicants because of infirmity, handcuffed into that position because their admissions policy required that all residents be able to carry on the tasks of daily living for themselves. Until the late 1970s, Poydras was not a "nursing home," as the term is commonly understood. However, in 1976, flush with financial assets, the board moved ahead with construction of an infirmary. This addition allowed the home to function as an intermediate care facility, sheltering women who, though initially admitted for independent living, had suffered declines of health and strength and needed greater assistance. The admission policy still required women to be able to care for their own needs upon entering, but the space designated "the infirmary" now existed to care for them if or when they declined. Though still a residence for ambulatory, elderly females who could pass a physical exam and gain approval from the board of managers for admission, Poydras Home offered a degree of nursing care after this expansion, so that aging residents would rarely be forced to leave to obtain greater levels of care. In addition to constructing a large, modern infirmary, the home added more residents' rooms and designated all of this new space as the John David Fink Memorial Wing.

Approaching the late twentieth century, the Poydras Home, with an enviable balance sheet, stood poised for a literal transformation of both its physical structure and its population, a transformation that the unpaid women of the board envisioned and then guided to completion. With means at hand, the managers embarked on a serious and time-consuming reevaluation of their mission. Their approach was thorough, grounded in serious study of demography, actuarial data, the literature of geriatric care, and every possible financial angle, including their investment portfolio, tax situation, real estate holdings, and current and proposed expenses. The demographic projections were starkly clear; the nation's elderly population was increasing dramatically. By the early 1980s, Americans over age sixty-five outnumbered teenagers for the first time in the country's history. Of interest to the Poydras managers was the dramatic increase in numbers of frail elderly who were functionally impaired but medically stable, seniors who required assistance with dressing, bathing, toileting, and/or mobility, and who would progress inexorably toward greater dependence. This was not the population Poydras had set out to serve when the conversion from children's home to retirement home was undertaken, but demographic data indicated that this was a rapidly growing population that needed help. At issue was what to do about it.

By 1994 the managers had hatched a hugely ambitious plan called Project '95, which, as things turned out, would not be completed until 1997, and which would demand massive expenditures. The goal was to upgrade and renovate existing space to better serve current Poydras residents and to expand the home's capacity to care for more highly dependent seniors in the future. The original orphanage that the Poydras Home occupied, coupled with additions and renovations, presented a handsome "street face," but, in fact, underneath a pleasing façade, time and use had taken a severe toll on the mechanical systems of the facility. Stopgap repairs had become a way of life. Physical plant supervisor Donald Dunn regularly tackled problems with the balky heating system, the ancient plumbing, an antiquated electrical system, inadequate air conditioning, and a seemingly endless series of leaks in the roofs. Project '95 would execute extensive renovations of all mechanical systems, upgrading electrical and plumbing, installing new heating and cooling systems, adding new security and fire alarms and a new copper roof. In addition, the project would add a new kitchen and chapel and expand Poydras to fifty-four beds, renovating some existing spaces to provide top-quality care for residents designated "highly dependent."

With Project '95, invigorated, ambitious managers committed themselves wholeheartedly to mastering the latest information about "best practices" in geriatric care. They began holding working retreats, intense overnight sessions at which they exchanged information, debated policy, and brainstormed nonstop. A delegation of board members regularly attended the annual national conferences of the American Association of Homes and Services for the Aging (AAHSA), where they faithfully went to sessions, asked questions, collected brochures, and took notes. They visited several highly regarded eldercare facilities in the South to observe what worked. For consultation, they brought in Dr. Lorraine Hiatt, a highly regarded, New York–based psychologist and gerontologist with vast experience in designing facilities for eldercare. Attentive managers attended her workshop and deemed it immensely useful. They listened as she explained that the crucial role of morning care in comfort and well-being necessitated having bedrooms that were private and spacious, with ample storage and private toilet rooms. Cautioning that reliance on diapers was not healthy, she explained the necessity of hiring more certified nurses' assistants for help with toileting, hygiene, and skin care. Hiatt commended the fact that Poydras served meals not on plastic trays but on china, at linen-spread tables, and urged the managers to continue the practice in a separate dining room for the highly dependent, recommending a separate activity room for this population as well.

The managers scribbled notes on all that Hiatt said. As the planning went forward, manager Mary Langlois, co-chair of Project '95, requested that the board consider three fundamental questions: "What are the things about Poydras Home we never want to change? What things definitely need changing? What would you hate to see happen to Poydras?"[13] Their chosen architect, E. Eean McNaughton, engaged in intense collaboration with Langlois and others in order to understand who they would serve at Poydras and how they wished to serve them. The managers insisted that the dependent-living arrangements were to be fitted out with the best and most appropriate devices and equipment, which they had learned about in their sessions and reading; at the same time, they assigned a high priority to attaining for each room the personal, noninstitutional environment that had always prevailed at the Poydras Home for the Elderly.

While Langlois spearheaded the design aspects of Project '95, board member Karen Gleye Smith was designated to manage the financial side, a tremendous and complex responsibility. The project's plans carried a price tag of between five and six million dollars. Four possibilities for financing such an expensive undertaking existed: traditional financing via a loan, paying cash by liquidating assets in the investment portfolio, paying cash by selling off sufficient real estate, or floating a nontaxable bond issue. Rounds of meetings ensued with bond specialists, investment counselors, bankers, and real estate agents as the managers gathered information before making a choice fraught with consequences.

Destiny took a hand in the fortunes of Poydras in the spring of 1995 when a fortuitous connection developed into a solution for financing Project '95. Representatives from the locally owned Whitney Bank approached the Poydras real estate committee about leasing an acre of the home's Magazine Street campus and building a branch bank there. Though not interested in this proposition, the managers seized the chance to meet face to face with King Milling and William L. Marks, the Whitney president and chairman of the board. At this first conference, managers Pat Rosamond and Karen Gleye Smith outlined Project '95 and indicated that they leaned toward selling state-issued nontaxable bonds as the preferred way to finance it. Repeated contact ensued, with the women providing detailed information about the financial standing and assets of Poydras. Ultimately, to the stunned delight of the board of managers, Whitney Bank offered to buy all the bonds itself. The managers then met to cast written ballots, indicating the gravity of the decision, on whether to accept the Whitney offer or to sell off assets and pay cash for the construction project. In the animated discussion preceding the balloting, a vocal and reluctant minority expressed fears regarding taking on long-term indebtedness, but in the end, near unanimity prevailed; only two managers voted against the Whitney bond option.

Managers traveled to Baton Rouge, met with the state bond commission, and won approval for issuing up to six million dollars' worth of bonds, under the auspices of the Health Education Authority of Louisiana (HEAL). The bonds were tax-exempt and had a maturity of fifteen years. Poydras was required to begin repaying its debt to Whitney Bank six months after issuance of the bonds. As security, they put up their rich portfolio of investments, but Whitney added a proviso that, should the value of stocks fall, always a possibility, the bank could require the managers to mortgage the home itself.

As the women made the choice to undertake such a gigantic project, treasurer Susan Kartzke admonished the managers to be particularly mindful of incurring expenses. Implementing a new but necessary policy, she warned that "no one should authorize or approve monies to be spent without checking first." Consumed with the consequential details of designing and financing Project '95, Mary Langlois and Karen Gleye Smith received a warmly supportive letter from the entire board, stating that they were "aware that you two are accomplishing the board's most important work right now . . . that you confront issues that interrupt your sleep . . . that you are required to consider decisions the potential outcomes of which are awesome." Expressing "much confidence in your ability to guide us," the letter closed with a promise. "We give you our thanks and we pledge you our support."[14]

Groundbreaking ceremonies occurred on March 14, 1996, as proud managers turned earth with ceremonial shovels and residents applauded; thereafter, construction proceeded in earnest. The elderly residents remained in the home throughout the construction, enduring noise and disruption with good grace. As a morale builder, the managers issued a plastic hard hat to every woman and encouraged all to observe the activities as much as they liked, which they did. Indeed, it became a point of fond teasing that many residents very much enjoyed watching the shirtless construction workers laboring at the site and bantering with the men. When the project concluded in late 1996, the genial workers reciprocated by inviting all the Poydras residents and managers to a barbecue on the grounds. To the immense pride and relief of the managers, the entire project came in under budget despite necessary change orders, owing to their relentless and competent monitoring of expenses.

Project '95 was but one of a series of changes at Poydras, significant changes that came thick and fast in the late twentieth century. Managers in the late 1980s had amended their constitution and bylaws, at last excising the words that mandated that residents be "white Protestant females," substituting simply "the elderly." This change opened the way not only for Catholics, Jews, and women of any race, but also for the admission of men, a highly controversial move discussed for years before finally occurring in the late 1990s. Going further, the board revised the mandate that none but Protestant women serve as managers and, in 1992, elected Poydras's first Catholic manager of the twentieth century.[15]

The home hummed with activities as well-trained personnel came on staff to conduct daily exercise classes, art and music therapy, arts and crafts, religious services, and more. An impressive welter of programs offered stimulation and entertainment for residents at various levels of independence: book club, cooking projects, casino day, fashion show, travelogues, guest speakers, Mother's Day brunch, parties for all holidays and birthdays, happy hour, plus outings to the Audubon Zoo, the Aquarium, and local restaurants. The ambitious managers began publishing a newsletter, the *Poydras Promise,* and staging a highly successful annual art show and sale. In 1987, Poydras hired its first professional social worker, who provided invaluable assistance in meeting nonmedical needs of residents, hearing their worries, mediating conflicts, helping newcomers adjust to institutional living, and offering support to family members during illness. A few years later, the managers added a consulting psychiatrist to their staff. Dr. Kenneth Sakauye met with residents who requested sessions and also offered informative and tremendously helpful programs for staff on topics such as post-stroke behavioral changes, changes in self-esteem among the aging, and appropriate management of the stages of Alzheimer's disease.

Today, the cruel Alzheimer's disease ranks sixth as cause of death in the United States, and according to the Centers for Disease Control and Prevention, 42 percent of residents now in assisted-living facilities exhibit signs of dementia. It is a virtual certainty that everyone reading this page knows or has known someone afflicted with Alzheimer's disease. To their great credit, the managers of Poydras began to grapple with the problem of dementia decades before it became a national topic of conversation. In 1980, for example, minutes summed up a protracted meeting's discussion in these words: "We must determine what kind of an institution we are. Do we continue to keep senile, disruptive patients? Patients who scream upset other residents. We must decide. As long as we can manage them do we keep them here until they die? Or, if they don't fit, do they have to leave, as specified on our Admissions Agreement when mental illness occurs?"[16]

By the late 1980s, the admissions committee had identified a trend: applicants to Poydras tended more and more to be older and, accordingly, were exhibiting more signs of senile dementia. The future of aging indicated that most who applied would come only after an increasingly difficult and ultimately futile struggle to remain in their own homes. The managers paid for staff to attend in-service training on management of Alzheimer's symptoms.

After much study, in 1999 the long-range planning committee made a definite recommendation that Poydras construct a unit dedicated to the care of Alzheimer's patients. The home could care quite well for Stage 1 and Stage 4 Alzheimer's patients since, in the first stage, the individual still related to her surroundings and functioned reasonably well and, in the last stage, she was no longer ambulatory and did not require labor-intensive care. Having a small unit dedicated to Stages 2 and 3 would provide a desirable continuum of care in one facility. The realization of that idea was Hunter House, which opened in May 2001, offering Alzheimer's patients their own activity and dining space, an enclosed outdoor area for "wandering," rooms with space for personal belongings, and an impressive staff-to-resident ratio. Striving to create a homelike atmosphere, the managers hoped to make the inevitable progression of the disease as comfortable as possible for the resident.

Another change took shape in bricks and mortar when Garden House assumed its place on the campus in July 2001. Prompted by the growing trend toward "aging in place," and the competition from burgeoning local eldercare facilities Lambeth House, Christwood, and Woldenberg Village, the managers elected to create ten units for independent living. They built a mix of efficiency, one-, and two-bedroom units, offering a meal plan, housekeeping, daily monitoring, and nurse's visits in case of illness, to be occupied by ambulatory residents only. The addition of these two new structures, Hunter House and Garden House, at a cost of over two million dollars, allowed the Poydras Home to become certified as a CCRC, or continuing care retirement community, one of only five in the state of Louisiana. This designation indicated that Poydras provided for each stage of aging: independent living, assisted living, intermediate nursing care, total nursing care, and special care for dementia and Alzheimer's, all on one campus.

Change also could be detected in the staff at the home. Since the shift of mission to eldercare, the caliber of senior Poydras employees had always been sterling; loyal longevity among supervisory staff in the crucial positions of housekeeping, physical plant, nursing, human resources, and activities was the norm at Poydras, meaning turnover at the upper levels was rare. The individuals in these posts spoke readily of belonging to "the Poydras family" and praised their work environment. Among the workers with lower skill levels, however, dissatisfaction was, unfortunately, common. Despite having been told repeatedly by administrators and outside evaluators that morale was low and turnover high among less skilled staff members because of inadequate benefits, the managers delayed implementing changes in this area for years. However, the alarming labor shortage after Hurricane Katrina forced their hand. With adoption of a benefits package sufficiently generous to allow Poydras to compete for scarce human resources, turnover fell and morale rose.

At the top of the Poydras pyramid of employees stood the home's administrator. Since 1994, only two individuals have held that post. Scott K. Crabtree, a professional with eleven years of health-care management experience, took the reins shortly before Project '95 commenced. Board members frankly admitted that without his steady management through that trying time, they felt they could not have executed their ambitious expansion and renovation at all. As chief administrator, Crabtree regularized procedures tremendously, bringing much-needed system and order to the Poydras Home. With ample input from appropriate manager committees, he produced a new code for personnel. Clear and fair, this code, coupled with highly specific job descriptions for all positions, which he crafted, contributed to the improved morale among staff. He instituted small but meaningful gestures of praise, such as a festive luncheon to honor employees when state licensing inspectors found no deficiencies whatever out of a possible 750 items on a checklist. He wrote a new safety manual and fire plan, as well as codes for residents, disaster, and maintenance, and inaugurated orderly purchasing procedures. Crabtree proved to be particularly adept at monitoring pending legislation for any adverse impact it might have on the Poydras operation and mobilizing Poydras managers and their circle of contacts to oppose the same. He held board members in high regard, observing while in the throes of Project '95, "Your dedication and commitment are awesome. Your desire to learn and to position the Poydras Home for the future is amazing."[17]

The managers likewise were well satisfied with Crabtree's performance. With one exception, that is; they noted, with no sense of irony, that "he should work on his ability to accept guidance from the Board."[18] His predecessor, Dr. Gordon Whyte of Tulane University, who had served briefly in an interim capacity while the board conducted its search for a permanent administrator, had told the managers in no uncertain terms that they were "overly involved" in the home's daily operations and warned that their hands-on approach hindered the performance of an efficient administrator.[19] Letting go, backing away, and relinquishing the details of daily operation came slowly to the board members, so ingrained in them were the traditions of nearly two centuries of literal management of the home. But change was just ahead.

By the late 1980s, the board conducted much of its work in specialized committees, which then filed detailed written reports with the full board, meaning that board meetings were streamlined in comparison with past practice. Committees with responsibility for specific aspects of the home's needs met independently of the full board, never less than monthly, and since managers usually served on two or more committees, service to the Poydras Home continued to demand a significant commitment of time. With increasing professionalism, the managers of the 1980s and 1990s consciously sought to recruit future board members who possessed certain attributes and skill sets rather than merely reach out to congenial women with whom they were socially acquainted. A 1989 letter from a board member to the full board, nominating an individual for a term on the board, observed that the nominee, who had served in various civic endeavors and clubs, was "a proven leader, intelligent, articulate, and assertive." In 1996, another letter of nomination, this one putting forward a woman who was senior legal counsel for Chevron in New Orleans, explicitly advocated change. "We are fast approaching a new century. Fewer women will have abundant free time. It is incumbent on us, the present Board, to put in place a more flexible meeting and committee structure to accommodate the younger, professional women who can offer so much to our institution as we move forward."[20]

As Poydras concluded its second century, the board opted to style itself as a "board of trustees," not managers, the simple name change indicating a meaningful shift in operational approach from day-to-day management to strategic and long-range planning, a shift that was a long time in coming. The adjustment in board governance emphatically signified the changing role of women. Occupations represented on the board at that point included architect, attorney, marketing professional, business administrator, health care administrator, and financial professional. Most on the board of trustees were engaged in professional careers, and all had been employed in the work force prior to joining the Poydras board. Spending the work day focused on legal briefs, spreadsheets, or real estate closings left little time for board members to devote to the quotidian inner workings of the institution for which they held broad fiduciary responsibilities and policy-making duties. Managers made the shift to rely on the professionalism of a competent administrator and his well-qualified team of staff members to make Poydras the institution they wanted it to be, day in and day out. The revolution in women's lives, brought about by the second wave of feminism, indisputably left its mark on the functioning of the Poydras board, whether individual managers called themselves feminists or not, and each trustee today approaches board responsibilities prepared by her professional as well as her personal experiences.

John S. "Jay" Rivé became executive director and CEO at Poydras upon the 2004 departure of Scott Crabtree, who was hired away by a New Orleans competitor, the continuing care retirement community of Lambeth House. Like his predecessor, Rivé, an experienced health care administrator, manifested high regard for the board members, and they for him. Their mutual admiration was fired in the crucible of Hurricane Katrina, one of the most unforgettable episodes in Poydras's two hundred years of service.

In the summer of 2004, the approach of powerful Hurricane Ivan had led Mayor Ray Nagin to call for a voluntary evacuation of the city.[21] After evaluating the situation soberly, Rivé addressed the Poydras residents whom he had gathered in the principal dining room. When he announced that they would be sheltering in place rather than evacuating, the room erupted in cheers. Chiefly native New Orleanians, the elderly residents had lived through decades of storms from the Gulf, including the destructive Betsy in 1965, and running away simply did not figure in their approach to hurricanes. As it happened, Ivan turned eastward and spared New Orleans anything more than heavy rain and some wind. However, it reinforced a narrative that told locals "the big one" was coming for them, if not this year, then sometime soon.

Earlier in the summer of 2004, the National Weather Service, FEMA, and Louisiana officials had executed a mock hurricane exercise, positing a fictional slow-moving, category 3 Hurricane Pam that hit New Orleans. The subsequent grim analysis of the drill indicated the likelihood of great destruction, massive displacement of people, and alarming death tolls. Having absorbed the recommendations promulgated in the wake of the Pam drill and follow-up, and then having had a close call with Ivan, Rivé updated his disaster plan for Poydras. He signed a contract with a local motor carrier; should he ever choose to evacuate his population, he wanted a written guarantee of bus service for the home's residents. He reached an agreement with a nursing home in Baton Rouge, some seventy-five miles upriver, to shelter Poydras residents at the Ollie Steele Burden Manor for the few days an evacuation of the city might require. He met with senior staff to explain what would be required should an evacuation of the home ever be deemed necessary. And then, having done all that seemed prudent, he, the residents, and the staff put disaster planning out of their minds.

The tropical storm season of 2005 was unusually active. In late August of that year, another mass formed over the southeastern Bahamas, gathered strength, and within days had gained the velocity to be named Katrina. The storm approached the southern tip of Florida early on Thursday, August 25, as a modest category 1 system, but immediately began to grow. Feeding off the superheated tropical waters, it accelerated across the Gulf of Mexico to menace the Gulf coasts of Louisiana and Mississippi. On Saturday, August 27, New Orleans awoke to the news that Katrina was already a category 4 storm, with miles of open water still to cross, making it nearly certain that she would become even more lethal. Landfall was predicted for early Monday morning, August 29. The "big one" was knocking at the door.

After evaluating the situation anxiously throughout that Saturday morning, administrator Rivé addressed the Poydras residents whom he had again gathered in the principal dining room. As in 2004, he announced that they would be sheltering in place rather than evacuating, and again the room of nervous elders erupted in cheers. Their life experience dictated that when hurricanes approached, one checked supplies of batteries and candles, laid in sandwich makings, iced down the beers, filled the bathtubs with water, secured outdoor furniture, then closed the shutters and waited.

Although gratified by the hugs and hurrahs with which residents showered him, a worried Rivé, also a New Orleanian, continued monitoring events. Scheduling a news conference, the state's governor, Kathleen Blanco, traveled to New Orleans on Saturday afternoon to exhort locals to leave the city ahead of the swelling storm. Even as officials were strongly urging, but not yet ordering, evacuation of the city, Rivé concluded by late evening of Saturday, August 27, that his initial decision could not stand: the ordeal of evacuation would be necessary after all. He placed calls to his leadership team—the directors of plant operations, nursing, and social services—to inform them that they would conduct a total evacuation of the Poydras Home on Sunday morning.

More phone calls followed: to the bus company ("I'm counting on you— be there!" he barked); to Ollie Steele Burden Manor, the Baton Rouge facility that would receive his storm refugees; and to his dietary supervisor. With the vivid example of the 2004 evacuation of tens of thousands of motorists from New Orleans in his mind, Rivé knew that the 70-mile trek to Baton Rouge, or- dinarily a drive of little more than an hour, would likely be an all-day ordeal in gridlocked traffic; he wanted his residents fueled with an especially ample hot breakfast, and gave instructions for that. Then he tried, unsuccessfully, to get some sleep.

Connie Brown, a veteran RN who worked part-time at Poydras, staffing the dementia unit in Hunter House, happened to be on duty that weekend. Also a native of New Orleans, she had felt no particular danger as the weekend began; her family had traveled to a ball game across the state while Brown worked her usual shift. Rivé phoned late on Saturday night to request her to help the residents prepare for the trip. Sunday morning found her shuttling from room to room, handing out large plastic garbage bags and instructing the seniors to pack clothing for a trip of three days' duration. Mindful of space limitations on the buses, again and again she playfully wagged a finger and reminded them, "No suitcases." Brown felt a strong affection for her charges and understood that they worried about leaving various treasures. For one, it was jewelry; for another, shelves of cherished photos; for yet another, a new television set. Stronger than resistance at leaving possessions was reluc- tance to be uprooted from the security of the Poydras Home. Brown recalled, "Residents were not happy that we had to leave. They just didn't want to go." She confidently reassured everyone that they would be home, safe and sound, by the middle of the next week.[22]

From around the region and, indeed, around the country, alarmed sons and daughters flooded the Poydras phone lines on Sunday with inquiries about plans for protecting their parents as the monster storm roared toward New Orleans. Senior staff patiently explained the evacuation plans to distant family members in the hours before departure. While they wielded phones, longtime physical plant supervisor Donald Dunn and his crew wrestled mat- tresses off beds, rolled them as tightly as possible, and crammed them into the wells of the two 55-passenger buses that had arrived for the mission. Others hurried to tie and label each resident's green garbage bag full of clothing and toiletry items. Still others labored to pull medical charts and count out appropriate dosages of medications for what all expected would be an interlude of three to four days in Baton Rouge. Jay Rivé described the harried efforts as "controlled chaos."

At last it was time for the frail residents to board the hulking buses that waited on the summer pavement rippling with noonday heat. While some climbed up unassisted, the many who leaned on walkers or relied on wheelchairs found themselves unable to execute the four steps up onto the big motor coaches. Strapping members of New Orleans Fire Company #5, whose engine house was only a short distance down the street, came to help the Poydras staff and, one by one, the seniors were lifted, carefully carried down the narrow aisles, and settled as comfortably as possible. Many staff members boarded to accompany their charges to their temporary home, and, with Connie Brown smiling and waving good-bye, having assured her beloved elders, "I'll see you next weekend," the buses pulled out with their reluctant human cargo, a caravan of Poydras employees following behind in their own cars and the home's van.

Some seventy miles and nine hours later, they reached their destination.

In the sweltering heat, the Poydras procession had bumped and inched its agonizingly slow way up Airline Highway, past countless overheated vehicles whose distressed operators abandoned them on the roadside, through gridlocked traffic that was at a total standstill for long minutes at a time. A city of nearly half a million people in flight had filled the highway beyond its capacity. Sharon King, veteran head of housekeeping, remembered that when the buses at last arrived, near dark, exhausted residents had to be carried off the vehicles. "We did it as a team, men and women; the ones who couldn't walk off, we toted 'em off."[23] Their stopping place was Ollie Steele Burden Manor, a trusted eldercare facility in Baton Rouge affiliated with the venerable Our Lady of the Lake Hospital. The nursing home boasted a new wing intended for Alzheimer's patients, just constructed but not yet occupied. Into that fortuitously empty space went the frail, weary Poydras refugees, bedded down on the floors on their own mattresses from the Poydras Home. Hurricane Katrina would make landfall early the next morning, while they slept.

The initial early morning bulletins brought good news to the anxious Jay Rivé, watching television in the pearly gray light of Baton Rouge: not only had the storm lost power; it had also changed its course. Rated a moderate category 3 when it came ashore at 6:10 a.m. on Monday, August 29, Katrina still packed sufficient force to obliterate the fishing and shrimping villages of Buras and Empire below New Orleans. From the mouth of the Mississippi River, however, Katrina tracked in a slightly northeasterly direction, ruinously smashing the coastal communities of Mississippi but miraculously sparing the Crescent City. Relieved people from New Orleans turned away from television screens to remind each other at breakfast, "We dodged a bullet." And so it seemed for a few brief hours, until ominous reports began to come: water rising in the streets of New Orleans, long after the storm surge should have subsided. The mighty storm had driven the waters of the lakes surrounding the city into shipping channels (the Mississippi River Gulf Outlet and the Industrial Canal) and the narrow outfall canals, which exist to drain the city when massive pumps operate to remove heavy rainfall. Now the storm-driven water's terrific force in narrow conduits was overwhelming manmade protective structures. In *Breach of Faith: Hurricane Katrina and the Near Death of a Great American City,* author Jed Horne offered a memorable and accurate description of just what happened.

> The surge sloshed higher and harder, bursting into the Industrial Canal with the force of a water cannon that... blew down the concrete flood walls ... and sent a Niagara of water thundering onto the streets and through the doors and windows and cracks in the houses.... The rising water in those drainage canals shoved aside levees and the concrete flood walls that had been added above them for an extra margin of protection. . . . It would never be known exactly how many people died. The best estimate placed the toll at about 1,100.... men, women and children attempted to wade or swim to dry ground, perched on rooftops awaiting help that never came, or succumbed to infernal temperatures and dehydration in attics where the floods had chased them.[24]

News coverage broadcast memorable images of the unforgivable suffering of refugees who took shelter in the Superdome, as instructed by the mayor.

The nation watched in shocked fascination as chaos ensued across the stricken city waiting for help, which was unfathomably slow to come. Gradually over the next hours and days, the true long-term horror of the situation became clear. New Orleans, famously below sea level, was catastrophically flooded and would remain so until pumped out (or "dewatered," as the Corps of Engineers insisted on terming it), a process that would take at least a month. Tens of thousands of homes were destroyed, many more badly damaged. The city's aged infrastructure for water and sewerage was simply wrecked. The utility company Entergy estimated it would need months to restore electric power, while the postal service reckoned on half a year for resuming home mail delivery. What had begun at the Poydras Home as a three-day excursion to safety in Baton Rouge became a hegira of open-ended, uncertain duration. Like Blanche DuBois, Poydras would now depend upon the kindness of strangers.

Caring staff members had willingly evacuated to Baton Rouge with the residents, a willingness predicated on their well-developed sense of duty. Housekeeper Sharon King said simply, "I left with the job." Some employees took young family members with them, on the expectation that the sojourn would be of short duration. When the predicted few days stretched into weeks, and ultimately into more than two months, strains inevitably developed. Poydras staffers slept in a recreation room at Ollie Steele, a communal accommodation that was the best that could be arranged at the time, and shared a nearby apartment in which to shower. Rivé realized that his workers needed private housing in Baton Rouge, to get them out of the makeshift arrangements offered by Ollie Steele Burden, but to his dismay, he discovered that FEMA had snapped up nearly all the available rental units for its own personnel. Adding to the tensions was the unexpected issue of childcare. Very young, often disruptive children of aides needed supervision while their mothers worked, but exhausted, dislocated workers, taking long shifts in an unfamiliar setting, understandably often did not fancy babysitting other women's children as one of their duties.

By the third or fourth day of unscripted life in makeshift quarters, some Poydras residents began to grow querulous. When Jay Rivé spoke by phone with one of the Poydras board members, she asked what he needed in Baton Rouge. His reply came immediately: "We need happy hour!" Indeed, the custom of serving glasses of wine every day at five o'clock was a longstanding practice at the Poydras Home.[25] Rivé intuited that its institution during the emergency would boost morale, and he was correct; pleasures of the grape helped everyone to bear less-than-ideal temporary arrangements. But the inescapable fact remained that Poydras was closed and no one knew when, or even if, it could reopen.

Back in the city, rock-steady employee Donald Dunn had stayed on the premises of the Poydras Home throughout the storm and subsequent flood. Dunn's wife and family sheltered at the home with him while he kept the emergency generator running, ensuring that the perishables in the big refrigerators were safe and the icemaker produced a plentiful supply of ice. As security, he gave his two pets, a Rottweiler and a chow, the run of the fenced property; both were good barkers but also his babies, gentle as lambs. Because of Poydras's situation on relatively high ground (the famous "sliver by the river"), the facility experienced no flooding; Poydras interiors were spared the muck and filth that filled so many New Orleans structures.

The sense of security did not last, however. On Tuesday, Dunn's adult daughter reported that the family home in the St. Roch neighborhood had collapsed; standing in water up to her shoulders, she had viewed it from afar. Dunn borrowed a bicycle the next day to see for himself, but returned to Poydras shaken by his outing. He saw a dead body, a frail form lying uncovered and defenseless at the corner of Magazine and Jackson Streets, only blocks from the Poydras Home. Aggressive local policemen stopped him and made it clear that they viewed him, an adult African American male on a bicycle, as someone who was trying to steal or burglarize unattended property. In broad daylight and without provocation, one officer pointed a pistol directly at Dunn and threatened to shoot him. "That kinda scared me," he remembered softly.[26] Back at Poydras, his family departed to seek sanctuary elsewhere, leaving him alone in the eerily deserted buildings. When his supply of diesel for the generator ran out, he flagged a National Guardsman to ask for help in getting more, to no avail. Days passed, but no one came to the home to check for survivors or to offer assistance. At week's end, Jay Rivé phoned; miraculously, although cell towers had toppled, the land lines at Poydras still functioned. He asked Dunn to bring the hard drives from Poydras computers so that they could tackle the process of issuing pay checks. Dunn locked up tight and left the Poydras Home for Baton Rouge.

Dunn was not the only Poydras staffer with a flood-destroyed home. Rivé's house in Old Metairie took water up to the ceilings and, like Dunn's, was uninhabitable. Thus, even as they struggled to keep the Poydras Home functioning in temporary quarters, as they worried over an eventual return to their Magazine Street property, Dunn, Rivé, and many other Poydras employees coped with their own heavy personal losses. In the short run, they needed to find temporary rental housing for their own families. Then they pivoted to face the protracted ordeal of dealing with claims adjusters, contractors, lenders, and the impenetrable bureaucracy of FEMA officialdom, all the while trying to concentrate on the comfort and well-being of the more than seventy bewildered old women and men who called Poydras home.[27]

After consulting as best he could with far-flung Poydras board members during the first two weeks of the crisis, Rivé began handing out pink slips to many of the home's employees. The facility at Ollie Steele Burden Manor had its own adequate staff of cooks, housekeepers, and custodians. As it became clear that the temporary evacuation would stretch out to fill weeks or maybe months, many family members came to Baton Rouge to retrieve their elderly relatives. Thus, the Poydras resident population declined, so that fewer nursing staff were needed. Each terminated worker departed with a month's severance pay and Rivé's instructions to keep in touch; as soon as Poydras could reopen, they would again be needed. But there were tears. The process was a painful ordeal.

In Baton Rouge, Rivé set up an office in a small room at the host facility from which he tried to project an air of normalcy in highly abnormal times. After several days, a blunt conversation with the administrator at Ollie Steele Burden convinced Rivé that he must place some Poydras residents elsewhere for the duration of the crisis. He found a nursing home in the little Acadian town of St. Martinville to take in the dementia patients, who required a great deal of nursing care; the remainder of the Poydras contingent stayed in Baton Rouge even though their presence at Ollie Steele caused some problems and friction. Throughout the crisis, Rivé was extremely reluctant to separate his population by sending two here and three there, as some at Ollie Steele had urged. He rejected finding temporary placements for his residents in scattered facilities because he frankly feared that those dispersed to faraway institutions might never return to a reopened Poydras if they lost their sense of belonging to the Poydras community, a sense they retained if kept together. And, always in his mind was the unspeakable nightmare scenario: if enough Poydras residents failed to return, the Poydras Home itself might fold, bringing to an end over 188 years of continuous service. Accordingly, he did all he could to ensure that those caught up in the Poydras diaspora still felt like Poydras family no matter where they lived. Several times a week, Poydras personnel drove the 120-mile round trip to St. Martinville to check on their residents personally, not only a morale builder but also an important ingredient in their getting good care.

Mercifully, by early October, some of the uncertainties began to lift. The despised Army Corps of Engineers (despised because universally blamed for faulty design and construction of the flood protection system that had failed so catastrophically) had at last "dewatered" the city by late September. It was possible to begin to evaluate and plan for return. Earlier, relying on nurse Connie Brown's Red Cross credentials, Rivé had driven through National Guard checkpoints with her to enter the blockaded and deserted city, surveying the damage firsthand. Now Rivé set a goal of having his staff back at work at the old home at ten o'clock on October 10, "ten-ten-ten," as they called it, to ready the premises for the ultimate goal, the return of the resident population from their enforced exile.

Where to find adequate staff loomed as the biggest question mark. Although Rivé had informed all Poydras employees that he would hold their positions for them until December 31, he soon learned that fully two-thirds of the pre-Katrina work force had refugeed elsewhere; conditions in New Orleans meant that they had no plans to return anytime soon. Regretfully, the absent workers had explained that the dearth of rental housing and functioning schools in New Orleans made it impossible for them to come back. He needed registered nurses, practical nurses, nurses' aides, kitchen assistants, and housekeepers, but the city's pre-Katrina population of over 450,000 had shrunk to around 150,000 in the fall of 2005, and the labor pool had diminished proportionately. In early October, Rivé ordered twenty signs reading simply NOW HIRING / POYDRAS HOME, with a phone number, and planted them at places that showed signs of life, such as the Walmart, the post office, and the ubiquitous Red Cross distribution centers. The response was positive and almost immediate. A full 20 percent of the city was unflooded, meaning that not every New Orleanian had lost housing. Rivé soon realized that he could hire highly qualified, reliable workers suddenly rendered jobless, though not homeless, because area hospitals where they had worked had closed after the destruction of the floods. The employment situation at Poydras was no longer a problem.

Employees came to work joyously on October 10, especially the Poydras veterans with flooded homes who had managed to find scarce rental housing in New Orleans. Poydras's suppliers were not yet delivering groceries in the crippled city, so Rivé had breakfasts, lunches, and suppers catered for his staffers, whose herculean task was to make the home as good as ever in three short weeks. Before reopening, Poydras would face rigorous mandatory inspections by various entities because it had suffered structural damage from winds and because the generator had shut down for lack of fuel. All employees worked long hours, scrubbing, sanitizing, painting, doing all that was necessary to create a clean, comfortable home for their displaced elders. There were outdoor tasks as well, clearing the debris and fallen trees and cutting tall grass to render the generous campus safe and lovely once again. There was much work to do with patient medical records, many of which had been lost during the evacuation when a Poydras van carrying charts and medications overheated and had to be abandoned by the roadside between New Orleans and Baton Rouge. Nurse Connie Brown laughed when she recalled the quantities of narcotics left behind in the vehicle and considered how New Orleans was allegedly swarming with ne'er-do-wells prowling the pharmacies and hospitals hoping to steal drugs in the chaotic hours after Katrina struck. "Narcotics beaucoup in there," she smiled, remembering the expired van.

Finally, the appointed day of November 1 arrived, and with it, the more than forty Poydras residents from Baton Rouge. There were tears on both sides as staff welcomed their charges back to the sanctuary of the Poydras Home. Head of housekeeping Sharon King, whose own elderly mother had sought shelter in a Canal Street hotel and had then been removed to the nightmares of the Superdome, recalled their gratitude. "It made you feel like family," she said. Donald Dunn echoed her memory. "Oh man, stepping off that bus was like getting off the plane to paradise. This was their home. They were so glad to be here." The shock of new faces in place of old familiar ones posed an initial challenge for many elders who were puzzled to find unknown aides coming to their assistance, but gratitude made them resilient. They were *home*.

Two weeks later, on November 15, the departure of twenty-two patients from the nursing home in St. Martinville signaled that the last contingent of scattered Poydras residents was headed back to familiar quarters. The caring St. Martinville staff had washed and set everyone's hair and packed sack lunches for all. Many townspeople turned out to wave good-bye to their guests from New Orleans. As the bus pulled out, leaving behind the little Cajun town tucked on the banks of Bayou Teche, Poydras residents and staff waved back, bringing to a close the Katrina exile from the Poydras Home.

Fewer than half of the nursing homes in the New Orleans area had evacuated as Katrina approached. Their owners and operators had resisted the increasingly alarmed pleadings of city and state officials, who implored locals to get out of the city; instead, they opted to shelter in place. Factors both humanitarian and financial must have influenced those decisions. Administrators worried over the capacity of their frail, elderly charges to survive a prolonged and strenuous evacuation in the heat of August, and it appears that some also worried over the price tag of executing such an endeavor. When the levees and floodwalls fell, waters rose with frightening speed throughout the city. Electric power failed, posing a danger for people dependent on oxygen machines and also for medically stable but weak elders whose bodies could not withstand the mega-heat of life without air conditioning. In the turbulent conditions developing in New Orleans, some rattled caregivers deposited elders at the shelter of last resort, the undersupplied, ill-equipped Superdome. Indelible images of suffering men and women, frail bundles of humanity slumped in their wheelchairs on the curb, unattended and alone in the blazing heat, were slow to fade from memory.[28]

In homes that did not evacuate before the storm, people died. Twenty-two died at the Lafon Nursing Facility run by the Sisters of the Holy Family, an African American order; nine of the Bethany Home's forty-nine residents died. Neither home had elected to evacuate. More horrific still were news stories of events at St. Rita's, a nursing home in the extremely low-lying parish of St. Bernard, a suburb just southeast of New Orleans. The owners, alone among the operators of five nursing homes in that parish, had chosen not to comply with a mandatory evacuation order. The comments of Gene Alonzo, a retired fisherman who saved his disabled brother there, sum up the scene that unfolded after Katrina came ashore and a towering storm surge inundated the building, flooding rooms up to the ceilings within twenty minutes. "In every room, people were hollering. They were screaming like somebody was murdering them. . . . It was a horror scene [until] . . . we just didn't hear no more screaming, no more calling for help." Although twenty-four residents were rescued by staff members, thirty-five helpless people drowned there, in their beds.[29]

Before the storm, Maison Hospitaliere and Pratt-Stanton Manor were trusted, well-established homes for the elderly in New Orleans. During the prolonged evacuation period in 2005, they dispersed their resident populations to various facilities across the region. Many of their shaken, exhausted elders opted to remain in the facilities where they had found refuge, and, consequently, Maison Hospitaliere and Pratt-Stanton never reopened. Living out Jay Rivé's nightmare scenario, they rank among the financial victims claimed by Katrina.

Rivé emphatically labeled the experience of Katrina "the hardest thing I've ever had to accomplish, *in my life*." Seventy-four Poydras residents were evacuated in August, and seven of them did not survive their difficult period of dislocation in Baton Rouge and St. Martinville. But Rivé's steadiness, coupled with a dedicated staff and a devoted board, brought the Poydras Home successfully through the crisis; together, they revived the facility so that it could go on. Like most New Orleanians, the board of managers spent much of the fall of 2005 in exile, scattered around the country. In November 2005, improving conditions in New Orleans allowed them to meet for the first time since Katrina. They quickly adopted a resolution to express their deepest gratitude to their homeless administrator, noting that he had "endured extraordinary personal sacrifice in his dedication to the residents of Poydras Home, directing all his energies to their care, comfort, and safety during their exile from the city of New Orleans." They saluted him because he led "by example." Appreciation assumed tangible form twice, first when managers voted handsome bonuses to Rivé and his employees, and again when the residents contributed $10,000 to the employees' Christmas fund and the board voted to match it.[30]

A much-cited cliché maintains that a crisis is a terrible thing to waste. The Katrina crisis certainly impressed lessons on Poydras managers and staff, who would face future storms much better prepared to deal with them. In fall 2005, Rivé elected to promptly pay the bus company that had ferried his population to Baton Rouge, rather than wait to collect promised FEMA money, as many did before addressing their storm-related bills. He wanted to ensure goodwill so that, in case of future need, he could be certain of buses and bus drivers at his disposal. Whitney Bank donated backpacks for each resident at Poydras, which now stand packed, labeled, and ready to go with a three days' supply of each resident's clothing and basic toiletries. Drug and medical records are computerized. The home purchased self-inflating air mattresses for all, which will be loaded into the buses along with the "hurricane bags," should another evacuation be necessary. The home runs an annual hurricane evacuation drill to ensure that all staffers and residents can execute plans for departure smoothly.

The post-Katrina annual report of the president of the board noted that Poydras was "bent by Katrina, but not broken." Revenue from properties declined for a time, but financial challenges had to be met. The fog of uncertainty was the biggest challenge as New Orleans struggled to rebuild. Unanswered questions troubled everyone in the city: When would buses and streetcars run again, and on which routes? Which schools would reopen, and when? When could shoppers again buy groceries in their own neighborhoods instead of driving ten miles to find a functioning suburban grocery store? When would mail delivery resume? Which hospitals would reopen? When would garbage again be collected on a regular basis? A particular challenge for Poydras concerned attracting and retaining quality employees in the competitive post-Katrina labor market. By 2006, the home offered generous salaries and benefits, but opportunities for work abounded in a situation of labor shortage. "Here at Poydras we are a bit like the ducks we see gliding calmly on the pond and paddling like crazy beneath the surface," president DeeDee Roussell commented, adding, "I am proud to be in this pond surrounded by such steady swimmers.

"One thing is for certain," Roussell continued, "Poydras Home will be a part of the rebirth of this city. Poydras has survived several yellow fever epidemics, the Civil War, two world wars, and numerous hurricanes, yet remains steadfast in its commitment to care and confident of its continued success in the future." Administrator Jay Rivé had echoed her sentiments when he welcomed tearful employees and residents back into the iconic old home in the fall of 2005. "This crisis is a minor speed bump in the evolution of Poydras," he told those assembled, as their hurricane exile came to an end. Voicing the attitude of the board of managers, he declared, "We are not going away!"[31]

As the Poydras Home approaches the milestone of two hundred years of continuous operation, the truth of those confident words is apparent. In 2013, yet another construction project was completed. Oak House is a three-story addition to the campus providing twenty-two spacious new assisted-living residences. One entire floor of this 27,000-square-foot addition functions to house residents in need of memory support. The changes include both new and renovated dining rooms, a spiritual and cultural center, and a well-appointed wellness and therapy gym. The facility now offers day care for elders, as well as residential services.

Determined to offer the best care possible for residents with dementia, board members continued to seek expert advice. In the months before the 2013 Oak House opening, the Poydras Home established a partnership with the Hearthstone Institute, an internationally recognized organization specializing in dementia care. Hearthstone professionals provided days of workshops on site so that staff assigned to Oak House could learn their philosophy and approach to dementia care, which places heavy emphasis on the unfailing recognition of people with dementia as individuals with emotional and psychological needs. Training everyone from top administrators to food and beverage workers in a non-pharmacologic approach to meeting the needs of people living with memory loss was a big, and rewarding, undertaking. Today residents in Oak House find encouragement to do what they enjoy, in a variety of Montessori-inspired activities always based on their individual likes and dislikes.

In the nineteenth century, a few long-lived managers seemingly wielded outsized influence at Poydras, but as of the twentieth, the work of Poydras managers had clearly become a genuinely collective effort. When the body became a board of trustees rather than managers, they also created the first Poydras Emeritus Board, starting with fourteen women who had each served ten years cultivating knowledge of Poydras. Their stellar contributions as active managers included the building of Garden House and Hunter House (facilities for independent living and Alzheimer's care), the inception of an adult daycare program and community outreach programs for Alzheimer's family support, the adoption of the new Poydras admissions policy, the creation of the first Poydras website (www.poydrashome.com), and, above all, Project '95, the momentous effort that really began the fundamental transformation of the Poydras Home. The first women inducted to the Emeritus Board were Dean Benko, Connie Dahlberg, Mary Demmas, Lois Downing, Catherine Edwards, Louise Ewin, Betsy Ewing, Kathleen Hobson, Mary Langlois, Susan McIntyre, Pat Rosamond, Nelda Sibley, Karen Gleye Smith, and Jeannette Smith. The board of trustees recognized that this group of veterans formed an extraordinarily rich resource of Poydras knowledge, dedication, and expertise. Emeritus status provided a way for current trustees to access both their institutional memory and their particular talents, even as the younger women eased the former managers into a less active role in governing their institution.

Though beloved former manager and board president Mabel Palmer chose not to take emeritus status because of considerations of health, her contributions were always warmly acknowledged. It was Palmer, a professional social worker of prominence in mental health circles in Louisiana, who instituted the first social worker position at Poydras, the first such position in a nursing home in New Orleans, and who saw the need for the services of a board-certified geriatric psychiatrist for counseling at the home. In short, her foresight changed Poydras substantially.

And now, as of this writing, an expanded and improved Poydras Home marches confidently into its third century, guided by the steady judgment of a committed, hardworking volunteer board, still composed of women only. Jay Rivé, who learned a thing or two about effort during the Katrina ordeal, observed emphatically, "I cannot tell you how impressed I am with their efforts."

The reader will perhaps recall the phrase "more durable than marble," which flowed from the articulate Mary Ann Hunter's pen in 1817 to laud benefactor Julien Poydras. How appropriate that she chose this metaphor. The reputation of Julien Poydras is, just as Hunter predicted, "more durable than marble." The Poydras Home itself is "more durable than marble." It only remains to say that the contributions of the members of the boards of managers, over long decades of service, are, likewise, "more durable than marble." No flashy or ostentatious description would fit their decidedly unglamorous work; we will not recall it as "more precious than rubies," as the poet sang in Proverbs, nor "more valuable than gold." No, the steady practicalities of Poydras managers (and now trustees) call to mind no substance so much as marble, a hard metamorphic rock whose characteristic veins and swirls are due to impurities in the mix, impurities that have been recast over time, by intense pressure, into a lovely, smooth, durable substance of great and lasting usefulness.

Two centuries have passed. A silver flute stoutly pipes a lovely but quiet melody. Other instruments join in, at first by ones and twos, then more and more. Steadily the melody grows and swells, until at last every instrument, in every section—brass, woodwinds, tympani, and strings—gives its all in a grand and powerful performance, polished and pleasing, emblematic of skill, commitment, cooperation, and professionalism.

And so the Poydras symphony plays on.

AFTERWORD

And so we see the effect of years of women's zeal on the institution they conceived, built, sustained, and expanded. But what of the effects of their activities on the women themselves? Service on the Poydras board of managers was essentially a career, a time-consuming and socially accepted extension of their designated roles as wives and mothers, giving them identities separate from their husbands. In the role of manager, women exercised executive skills, making policy, planning budgets, hiring and dismissing employees. From their very start in 1817, their actions had a political dimension; they approached state officials for an act of incorporation and later had frequent dealings with both city and state government.[1]

Before the institution of term limits for managers in the mid-twentieth-century constitution, women not uncommonly served on the Poydras board for decades. Meeting with her counterparts twice or more each month for hours at a time, each manager focused on protecting needy and neglected girls from the physical and moral dangers at large in New Orleans. Wrestling with nearly intractable problems of budget, personnel, or discipline, these women drew on their skills and personal resources to find solutions. Frequently decisions were not unanimous, but the women kept a serene equilibrium. They had their detractors; they incurred criticism. Twice in the first five years, the secretary mentioned this, noting that "the voice of ridicule . . . frequently assailed them" and ruefully recalling "smiles of contempt."[2]

Undertaking benevolent work together under such conditions fostered strong, warm bonds among these women. Though they retained a formality in their dealings with each other, there is no mistaking the genuine affection and regard that they felt. Resolutions inserted into the minutes upon the death of a "lady manager" make this clear. A lengthy and moving tribute to founding manager Ann Bryant upon her death in 1817 noted that her last visit from her home was to the asylum to see the girls. "Where is she now to whose counsel we used to listen with pleasure, and adopt from conviction?" they asked. Upon Phoebe Hunter's death in 1844, they recorded that she had "fanned into life the flame of benevolence that burned in the breast of the founders of this orphan asylum . . . our dear and respected Mrs. Hunter." On April 20, 1849, managers assembled in a called meeting to commemorate the life of "the venerable Mrs. Duplessis," whom their resolution described as "always ready, regardless of personal care, to serve the orphans and the widow," noting that "even when feeble health prevented her attendance regularly . . . her thoughts were with us . . . her heart was as warm and her ear as open to the sad appeal of the bereaved little ones as when in the years of her strength she plead [sic] for them at our Board." When Phoebe G. Laidlaw died in 1878, they reflected solemnly that they would "see her no more, no more be cheered by her placid and approving smile," and lauded "the beauty and strength of her character, her self-denying Christian heart, that gentle spirit of true charity that thinketh no evil ever, apparent in her bearing to all," concluding simply, "The loss is truly irreparable." Only a year later, they remembered the late Clemence Toby as "affectionate, unostentatious, modest . . . a sweet presence among us" and paid fond tribute to "her amiable character & forbearance . . . her active benevolence to relieve distress, being the ruling principle of her life." In 1881, the loss of Mary Luzenberg led the managers to pass similar resolutions upon her death ("the maturity of her judgment and firmness of character were combined with gentleness, kindness and uniform amiability") and to take the further step of printing them in the local *Picayune*. Though, as historian Anne Firor Scott observed of other women engaged in benevolent work, their recorded comments, couched in language derived from sentimental novels and the King James Bible, make them sound a bit like Marmee in *Little Women*, we have no reason to doubt that they possessed the sterling characteristics enumerated; such traits were the height of womanly virtue in that century.[3]

The changing times of the twentieth century put the women of Poydras through great difficulties. The very nature of benevolence had altered, as had the population they served. Adaptation was essential if their institution was to survive, and after some stumbles, they did adapt. They proved able to learn and to grow. Profiting from mistakes, taking risks, changing with the times, the women of Poydras prevailed. Confident and capable, they enter a third century, heirs to Phoebe Hunter's vision and sisters in spirit to the long line of managers who went before them.

NOTES

1. Orphans and Orphanages: A Historical Overview

1. Homer Folks, *The Care of Destitute, Neglected, and Delinquent Children* (New York: Macmillan, 1902), 29.

2. Information on the 1909 White House conference comes chiefly from Matthew A. Crenson, *Building the Invisible Orphanage: A Prehistory of the American Welfare System* (Cambridge, MA: Harvard University Press, 2009), 7–15.

3. Quoted in Theda Skocpol, *Protecting Soldiers and Mothers: The Political Origins of Social Policy in the United States* (Cambridge, MA: Belknap Press of Harvard University Press, 1992), 425.

4. Linda Gordon, *Pitied but Not Entitled: Single Mothers and the History of Welfare, 1890–1935* (New York: Free Press, 1994), 49–50.

5. Kenneth Cmiel, *A Home of Another Kind: One Chicago Orphanage and the Tangle of Child Welfare* (Chicago: University of Chicago Press, 1995), passim. I am greatly indebted to Cmiel's lucid outline of developments at Chapin Hall, which were replicated to some extent at the Poydras Home.

2. The Genesis of an Idea

1. Jefferson actually appointed three fact-finding missions beyond the well-known Lewis and Clark expedition: the Freeman-Custis expedition up the Red River, the Zebulon Pike expedition into the Rocky Mountains, and the Dunbar-Hunter expedition up the Ouachita River.

2. Quoted in Trey Berry, Pam Beasley, and Jeanne Clements, eds., *The Forgotten Expedition, 1804–1805: The Louisiana Purchase Journals of Dunbar and Hunter* (Baton Rouge: LSU Press, 2006), xiii.

3. Lawrence Powell, *The Accidental City: Improvising New Orleans* (Cambridge, MA: Harvard University Press, 2012), 296.

4. Quoted in Richard Campanella, *Bienville's Dilemma: A Historical Geography of New Orleans* (Lafayette: Center for Louisiana Studies, University of Louisiana at Lafayette, 2008), 167.

5. Quoted in Lawrence N. Powell, *The Accidental City: Improvising New Orleans* (Cambridge, MA: Harvard University Press, 2012), 217.

6. Quoted in Peter J. Kastor, *The Nation's Crucible: The Louisiana Purchase and the Creation of America* (New Haven: Yale University Press, 2004), 179.

7. Quoted in Margaret Hope Bacon, *The Quiet Rebels: The Story of Quakers in America* (New York: Basic Books, 1969), 78.

8. Berry et al., eds., *The Forgotten Expedition,* xxxiv.

9. Mark Duvall, "Phoebe Hunter, 1760–1844: Neither Northern nor Southern," in *Louisiana Women,* vol. 2, ed. Shannon Frystak (Athens: University of Georgia Press, forthcoming), 436–37. I am much indebted to Mark Duvall for so generously sharing his work in a prepublication stage. His valuable probing of Quaker records held at Haverford College in Pennsylvania illuminated Phoebe Hunter's pre–New Orleans background for me.

10. Rosemary Abend, "Constant Samaritans: Quaker Philanthropy in Philadelphia, 1680–1789" (Ph.D. diss., University of California Los Angeles, 1988).

11. Margaret Morris Haviland, "Beyond Women's Sphere: Young Quaker Women and the Veil of Charity in Philadelphia, 1790–1810," *William & Mary Quarterly* 51 (July 1994): 419–46, offers an excellent discussion of the pathbreaking benevolent activities of young Quaker women. The quoted passage is found on p. 429.

12. "The Late Mrs. Hunter," *New Orleans Commercial Bulletin,* January 8, 1844.

13. Bruce Dorsey, "Friends Becoming Enemies: Philadelphia Benevolence and the Neglected Era of American Quaker History," *Journal of the Early Republic* 18 (Autumn 1998): 400.

3. Humble Beginnings and a Generous Benefactor

1. Typescript, "History compiled for centennial 1917 by Miss Daisy Hodgson," Box 27, Poydras Home Papers; John Smith Kendall, *History of New Orleans,* vol. 2 (Chicago: Lewis Publishing Co., 1922), 644–45; Lillian Fortier Zeringer, "The History of Poydras Home" (N.p.: n.d. [c. 1977]), 8–9.

2. Secretary's annual report for 1831, January 16, 1832; minutes of April 25, 1837, and May 13, 1857, Poydras Home Papers. The Poydras Home also proudly displays a portrait of patron Julien Poydras. For years, it was believed that the artist was renowned painter Benjamin West. However, authorities at the New Orleans Museum of Art have determined that the painter who executed the likeness was actually William Edward West, who studied under Thomas Sully in Philadelphia. Minutes of January 4, 1962, Poydras Home Papers.

3. The women amended their constitution in 1821 to expand the board of managers from nine to twelve.

4. Theodore Clapp, *Autobiographical Sketches and Recollections: During a Thirty-Five Years' Residence in New Orleans* (Boston: Phillips, Samson & Co., 1857), 86.

5. Statement of purpose recorded on first page of original minute book (January 1817), Poydras Home Papers.

6. Quoted in Lori D. Ginzberg, *Women and the Work of Benevolence: Morality, Politics, and Class in the Nineteenth-Century United States* (New Haven: Yale University Press, 1992), 38.

7. Original constitution of Female Orphan Society, copied in minutes of January 21, 1817, Poydras Home Papers. Italics mine.

8. In order for women to retain property they brought to a marriage, however, a special antenuptial agreement was required, exactly as under English common law. Few first-time brides availed themselves of this mechanism; widows who planned a second marriage, having learned by experience, were more likely to take steps to protect their property for themselves and their heirs.

9. *A Digest of the Civil Laws Now in Force in the Territory of Orleans, With Alterations and Amendments Adapted to its Present System of Government* (New Orleans: Bradford & Anderson, 1808), Book I, Title IV, Chapter IV, article 21 ("Of the Respective Rights and Duties of Married Persons"). I am grateful to Mark Fernandez for offering useful insights about women and the law in early Louisiana.

10. Copy of act of legislature, recorded in minutes of March 1, 1817, Poydras Home Papers. Italics mine.

11. Minutes of February 1, 1817, Poydras Home Papers.

12. M. A. Hunter to Julien Poydras, February 1, 1817, Poydras Home Papers.

13. For details of the life of Julien Poydras, I have relied primarily upon Brian J. Costello, *The Life, Family and Legacy of Julien Poydras* (N.p.: John and Noelie Laurent Ewing, 2001).

14. Gwendolyn Midlo Hall, *Africans in Colonial Louisiana: The Development of Afro-Creole Culture in the Eighteenth Century* (Baton Rouge: LSU Press, 1992), 333.

15. Quoted in Christina Vella, *Intimate Enemies: The Two Worlds of the Baroness de Pontalba* (Baton Rouge: LSU Press, 2004), 19.

16. Hall, *Africans in Colonial Louisiana,* 364.

17. His townhouse address was 471 Bourbon Street, which later became the site of Owen Brennan's Vieux Carré, also known as "Brennan's," a longtime favorite among New Orleans restaurants. In 1956 Brennan's moved to 417 Royal Street.

18. The romantic exaggerations about Poydras's putative lost love gained extra circulation in 1941 when MGM released a "short" entitled *Strange Testament.* The story line conjured up a beautiful woman who so captivated the young Poydras when they met, amid the giddy possibilities of a Carnival ball, that he proposed marriage that very evening. However, he ungallantly abandoned his offer when he squired her home and discovered the conditions in which she lived. The short film improbably implied that the young gentleman had no choice but to walk away from a common girl who lived in poverty, but also maintained that his lasting heartache led him, years later, to provide for dowries for poor females in his will. Perpetuation of the myth continues; Turner Classic Movies screened *Strange Testament* in November 2015. See also http://www.imdb.com/title/tt0143908/ (accessed November 30, 2015).

19. Copy of announcement in minutes of March 8, 1817, Poydras Home Papers.

20. I am indebted to Mark Duvall for these statistics, which he compiled for his master's thesis, "The New Orleans Female Orphan Society: Labor, Education, and Americanization, 1817–1833" (M.A. thesis, University of New Orleans, 2009), 19.

21. Italics mine. The minutes show that the women on the Poydras board routinely referred to those living at the asylum as "the family." Minutes of February 22, 1817, contain a list of rules adopted for governing the newly established asylum; copy of managers' letter to Rev. Sylvester Larned in minutes of May 10, 1818, Poydras Home Papers.

22. Suzanne Lebsock, *The Free Women of Petersburg: Status and Culture in a Southern Town, 1784–1860* (New York: Norton, 1985), 205.

23. Secretary's annual report for 1817, January 21, 1818, Poydras Home Papers.

24. Paul LaChance, "The 1809 Immigration of Saint-Domingue Refugees to New Orleans: Reception, Integration and Impact," *Louisiana History* 29 (Spring 1988): 141; Mary Ann Hunter to Cousin Eliza, July 30, 1815, quoted in Duvall, "Phoebe Hunter," 434.

25. Secretary's annual report for 1817, January 21, 1818, Poydras Home Papers.

26. Ibid.

27. Minutes of January 10, 1817, Poydras Home Papers.

28. B. B. Edwards, *Memoirs of the Rev. Elias Cornelius* (Boston: Perkins and Marvin, 1833), 92.

29. The minutes record that, beyond the seven taken into the asylum itself, Phoebe Hunter and her daughter Phoebe G. Laidlaw each took a girl into her own home, possibly because the girls needed skilled nursing or more constant care than could be provided at the asylum, or more likely because they were the indentured servants and could labor in their households. Minutes of March 1, 1818, Poydras Home Papers.

30. Minutes of April 1822, Poydras Home Papers.

31. An elderly woman who lived in the asylum as a girl in the 1920s recalled that when the managers dined with them, the tables featured "ladies' butter," but, day in and day out, the asylum children did not routinely enjoy such a luxury. However, the existing records frequently mention butter as part of the nineteenth-century fare.

32. Minutes of August 7, 1823, January 15, 1829, and September 5, 1844, Poydras Home Papers.

33. For example, the managers responded negatively to a request by a Mrs. Torrence to have her daughters sent to her at an address out of town. "Whilst the Ladies appreciated your desire to have your children with you, in veiw [sic] of their comforts, where they are, and the entire absence of a home to which you could take them, being yourself without one, they unanimously decided that it would not be to the interest of your children to send them to you at this time. . . . it is best for your children to remain where they are." Undated draft of letter to Mrs. Torrence, Box 26, Poydras Home Papers.

34. Minutes of July 4, 1827; secretary's annual report for 1846, January 1847, Poydras Home Papers.

35. Minutes of October 2, 1823, Poydras Home Papers.

36. Minutes of September 20, 1855, Poydras Home Papers.

37. Minutes of July 19, 1838, and February 16, 1843, Poydras Home Papers.

38. Ruth Wallis Herndon and John E. Murray, eds., *Children Bound to Labor: The Pauper Apprentice System in Early America* (Ithaca: Cornell University Press, 2009), 2.

39. Legislative act recorded in minutes of June 5, 1819, Poydras Home Papers.

40. Minutes of March 3, 1836, Poydras Home Papers. Emphasis in original.

41. Minutes of April 5, 1817, Poydras Home Papers.

42. Minutes of February 17, 1817, and May 15, 1817, Poydras Home Papers.

43. Secretary's annual report for 1824, dated January 1825, Poydras Home Papers.

44. Emily Clark, *Masterless Mistresses: The New Orleans Ursulines and the Development of a New World Society, 1727–1834* (Chapel Hill: University of North Carolina Press, 2007), 229.

45. Minutes of October 5, 1821, Poydras Home Papers. The mayor referred to was Count Louis Philippe de Roffignac (1766–1846), the French-born soldier who emigrated to Louisiana in 1800 and served as mayor of New Orleans, 1820–1828.

46. Minutes of May 1, 1823, Poydras Home Papers.

4. Years of Growth

1. Their first stock purchase represented ten shares in the Louisiana Bank, of which their patron Julien Poydras was president.

2. Secretary's annual report for 1819, January 17, 1820, Poydras Home Papers.

3. Secretary's annual report for 1826, January 16, 1827, Poydras Home Papers. At the time of their decision about construction, the managers had assets of $2,500 in bank stock, a $2,000 appropriation from the state legislature, and $1,200 from the city, plus sundry lesser funds for operating expenses. The low bid for the new asylum was $6,200.

4. Minutes of February 17, 1825, and April 1, 1825, Poydras Home Papers.

5. Minutes of July 13, 1829, Poydras Home Papers.

6. Minutes of May 10, 1831, Poydras Home Papers. The women placed a value of $1,000 per year on this lot, but attorney Livermore urged them to take less. In July 1831, their auctioneer won a bid of $1,650, thus amply validating their rebuff of the lawyer's advice.

7. Minutes of April 4, 1839, May 16, 1839, September 7, 1839, and September 10, 1839, Poydras Home Papers.

8. Minutes of October 19, 1848, Poydras Home Papers. With properties received from esteemed benefactor Julien Poydras, they regularly leased but never sold. They leased the site of their original asylum, a particularly prime lot on St. Charles Avenue, for a period of fifty years to Dr. George W. Campbell, prosperous sugar planter and physician. Just before the outbreak of the Civil War, he erected an Italianate mansion there at the then-extravagant price of some $90,000 (exclusive of furnishings) and, soon afterwards, departed to serve as a surgeon for the Confederate troops. When General Benjamin Butler looked over the city for a properly elegant residence for himself and his lady during the Federal occupation, his eye fell upon Campbell's grand home. Pleased, the general claimed it for his own and unceremoniously evicted the doctor's wife and five children, provoking intense outrage among the civilian population of the city. The fact that the Campbells alleged considerable loss of personal property, including flatware, while their home was in the general's possession contributed to

his unflattering nickname "Spoons" Butler, which stuck at least as well as his other sobriquet, "Beast." Dr. Campbell's lease with the Poydras women gave him possession for fifty years, after which the lease might be renewed or the Poydras managers obligated to buy the structure Campbell had built. Judge Henry Spofford, a Louisiana Supreme Court justice, took over the lease for the house at 195 St. Charles Avenue from Dr. Campbell a few years after the war, but died in 1880. Here began the sad undoing of a once-dazzling residence, which enjoyed some years as a desirable boardinghouse but declined as the neighborhood around it changed drastically.

In 1907, Poydras managers wrote to Mayor Martin Behrman, complaining of the existence of "disreputable houses" in the vicinity of this property, to no avail. When the fifty-year lease expired in 1908, managers reclaimed the property, made some structural changes, and began operating the elegant old building as the Mansion House Apartments. Tenants seemed to inflict a great deal of damage there, however, necessitating frequent repairs, and the apartment house never yielded a significant profit. In 1965, impervious to requests from the Louisiana Landmarks Society to find a way to preserve such a historically significant building, the board of managers ignored a community outcry of opposition from outraged preservationists and razed the Campbell mansion. A parking lot now occupies the site. The carriage house to its rear avoided the wrecking ball, however, and survives to the present.

9. Secretary's annual report for 1838, January 16, 1839, Poydras Home Papers.

10. Secretary's annual report for 1851, January 16, 1852, and secretary annual report for 1853, January 16, 1854, Poydras Home Papers.

11. Secretary's annual report for 1852; minutes of January 17, 1853, Poydras Home Papers.

12. Minutes of April 21, 1853, Poydras Home Papers.

13. Secretary's annual report for 1854, January 16, 1855, Poydras Home Papers.

14. Secretary's annual report for 1857, January 16, 1858, Poydras Home Papers.

15. Quoted in Zeringer, "History of Poydras Home," 38.

16. Minutes of June 5, 1856, Poydras Home Papers.

17. The site of two squares of ground (approximately seven acres) was bounded by Magazine, Leontine, Laurel, and Peters Streets. Peters today is Jefferson Avenue.

18. Minutes of August 20, 1857, Poydras Home Papers.

19. Dr. J. Rhodes to "Lady Directors," July 7, 1853, Box 3, Poydras Home Papers.

20. The quote attributed to Margaret Haughery is from a little volume entitled *Margaret of New Orleans,* compiled and edited by "A Friend of the Family" and published in 1913. Poydras minutes of June 5, 1879, specifically report the purchase of bread at cost from Margaret Haughery. Reliable biographical information about Haughery comes from Laura Kelley's entry "Margaret Haughery" in *KnowLa Encyclopedia of Louisiana,* http://www.knowla.org/entry/790/&view=summary.

21. The women's appeal appeared in several local newspapers. This quotation comes from the *Louisiana Courier,* April 27, 1858.

22. M. Adams to Mrs. Luzenberg, President & Managers of the Poydras Asylum, May 10, 1858, Box 3, Poydras Home Papers.

23. S. Frederick Starr, *Southern Comfort: The Garden District of New Orleans* (New York: Princeton Architectural Press, 1998), 46.

24. The schoolroom teacher, Mrs. Nelson, had assigned the older girls to write a composition in the form of a letter to a friend or relative, telling the news of Mrs. Laidlaw's death. Box 27, Poydras Home Papers.

25. First quotation from obituary tribute of Rev. H. M. Smith, published in the *Southwestern Presbyterian,* according to minutes of a called meeting of the board, February 23, 1878; second quotation from typescript, "History compiled for centennial 1917 by Miss Daisy Hodgson," Box 27, Poydras Home Papers.

26. Quoted in Frances Jordan, "Poydras Asylum Celebrates 130th Year," *New Orleans States,* January 17, 1947.

27. A typical visitor's report is Mrs. Richardson's summary from November 12, 1862: "Pleased to see the infirmary empty—no sickness of any consequence on hand. Nursery noisy as usual but all comfortable under the care of a very kind nurse, tho' defective in energy and perhaps neatness. Sewing department in best condition of activity and order" (managers' notebook, November 12, 1862, Poydras Home Papers).

28. For example, when manager Estelle Hodgson died in May 1894, her daughter Daisy joined the board and served as secretary until her death in 1940. Longtime board member Clemence Toby was succeeded by her daughter Mrs. W. S. Campbell, who was in turn succeeded by her daughter, Mrs. Watts Leverich, making a total of nearly one hundred years' service from the three generations of that family. Mrs. O. J. Paul succeeded her mother Mrs. Howard Smith. In the late twentieth century, the tradition continued with Karen G. Smith succeeding her mother-in-law Charlotte Carter Smith and Stevia Walther following in the footsteps of her mother Marion Lifsey.

5. Crosses to Bear: The Impact of Religious Strife on the Poydras Asylum

1. Minutes of November 5, 1838, Poydras Home Papers.

2. Secretary's annual report for 1824; minutes of January 1825, Poydras Home Papers.

3. Minutes of February 17, 1825, Poydras Home Papers.

4. The minutes for May 19, 1825, specifically refer to Catholic managers. The affiliations of managers are not stated in the minutes, but one may infer that women with French names were likely Catholic. The managers were Phoebe Hunter, Celeste Duplessis, M. T. Chew, P. G. Laidlaw, Felicite Depeyster, Fidelite Polk, Felicite Foucher, A. M. Linton, S. H. Morgan, Sophia Kennedy, E. Stringer, and S. S. Hull.

5. Minutes of October 7, 1829, Poydras Home Papers.

6. Thomas G. Conway, "John A. Kennicott: A Teacher in New Orleans," *Louisiana History* 26 (Autumn 1985): 401.

7. Minutes of September 13, 1830, Poydras Home Papers.

8. Copy of Laidlaw's letter in minutes of September 13, 1830, Poydras Home Papers.

9. For an overview of the intensely heated dissension between Protestants and Catholics in the antebellum period, I have relied primarily on Ray A. Billington's classic study, *The Protestant Crusade, 1800–1860: A Study of the Origins of American Nativism* (New York: Rinehart, 1938).

10. Susan M. Griffin, "'The Dark Stranger': Sensationalism and Anti-Catholicism in Sarah Josepha Hale's *Traits of American Life*," *Legacy* 14 (1997): 15.

11. Richard Hofstadter, *The Paranoid Style in American Politics* (New York: Knopf, 1965), 22.

12. *New Orleans Picayune,* February 7, 1837, 2.

13. Billington, *Protestant Crusade,* 142.

14. Clement Eaton, *Freedom of Thought in the Old South* (Durham NC: Duke University Press, 1940), 299. Rev. Theodore Clapp (1792–1866) shepherded Sylvester Larned's Presbyterian Church in New Orleans until 1832. At that time, because of his growing doubts about Trinitarian doctrine and outright rejection of eternal damnation, the earnest and popular but highly unorthodox minister was ousted from his position. He continued to preach, however, founding a house of worship that he called the First Congregational Church, although it adopted Unitarian-Universalist theology. Through his ecumenical, liberal pulpit messages and his personal conduct, Clapp demonstrated "essential goodwill toward the Roman church." Many of his original congregation remained with him after the split, while others ("a remnant of hard-core Presbyterians") established the First Presbyterian Church of New Orleans. Phoebe Hunter's daughter and son-in-law Phoebe and Peter Laidlaw were among the leading followers of Clapp who clung to him after the schism in the First Presbyterian Church. Timothy F. Reilly, "Parson Clapp of New Orleans: Antebellum Social Critic, Religious Radical, and Member of the Establishment," *Louisiana History* 16 (Spring 1975): 177, 172.

15. Minutes of November 1, 1832; secretary's annual report for 1832, January 1833, Poydras Home Papers.

16. Both letters are from Sister Regina to Mother Augustine, her superior in Emmitsburg, Maryland; the first quotation is from correspondence dated January 12, 1833; the second is dated March 1833. Quoted in Sister Zoe Glenski, "The Work of the Daughters of Charity in New Orleans, 1830–1900" (M.A. thesis, Xavier University of New Orleans, 1959), 15–16, in Office of Archives and Records, Archdiocese of New Orleans.

17. Minutes of September 10, 1834, Poydras Home Papers.

18. Lydia Skinner to Lady Managers, November 27, 1834, Box 1, Poydras Home Papers.

19. Minutes of January 27, 1836, April 7, 1836, and April 15, 1836, Poydras Home Papers.

20. Minutes of June 16, 1836, Poydras Home Papers.

21. Minutes of May 5, 1836, Poydras Home Papers.

22. Minutes of June 28, 1836, Poydras Home Papers.

23. Minutes of September 11, 1836, Poydras Home Papers.

24. Minutes of February 6, 1832, copy of managers' letter to "Superiors of St. Joseph at Emmitsburg, Maryland," February 8, 1832, both in Poydras Home Papers; Sister Lorretta (S.C.), Donaldsonville, La., to Bishop A(ntoine) Blanc, New Orleans, November 30, 1847, in Office of Archives and Records, Archdiocese of New Orleans.

25. John O'Grady, *Catholic Charities in the United States: History and Problems* (Washington, DC: National Conference of Catholic Charities, 1931), 94.

26. Father Adam Kindelon, New Orleans, to "Dear Father" (Bishop Antoine Blanc), Lyon, France, July 8, 1836, in Office of Archives and Records, Archdiocese of New Orleans.

27. Minutes of October 25, 1836, Poydras Home Papers.

28. Minutes of November 4, 1836, Poydras Home Papers.

29. Ibid.

30. Minutes of December 19, 1836, Poydras Home Papers.

31. Secretary's annual report for 1836, January 16, 1837, Poydras Home Papers.

32. J. I. Mullen, R.S.P., to "My dear madam," January 20, 1848, Box 2, Poydras Home Papers. The description of Father Mullen comes from Charles E. Nolan, *Religion in Louisiana* (Lafayette LA: Center for Louisiana Studies, University of Louisiana at Lafayette, 2004), 430.

33. Minutes of February 3, 1848, and February 17, 1848, Poydras Home Papers. The struggle between Father Mullen and the Poydras managers reflected a difference in ideology. Many Catholics shared the priest's rejection of the Protestant view that life in a genuine but non-Catholic family was superior to impersonal institutional care for Catholic children. Indeed, spurning the model of foster care, which was often managed by Protestant groups or government agencies, Catholics continued to operate asylums well into the twentieth century, even as the practice declined generally. See Hacsi, *Second Home,* 72–74.

34. However, as with so much of life in the Crescent City, Know-Nothingism in New Orleans was unique, not like that phenomenon in the United States at large. Populated by many Creoles, the movement targeted foreigners, meaning chiefly Irish and German newcomers. Creoles had fretted over their diminishing importance in the city for decades, ever since the "American" influence began to rise early in the nineteenth century. Seeing that the new arrivals tended to identify with American values, Creoles viewed them as a threat because they increased the number of non-Creoles in New Orleans. Many of the city's Creoles initially embraced Know-Nothingism, drawn by its virulent nativism. In New Orleans, therefore, both the Know-Nothings and those they attacked were predominantly Catholic, a true oddity in a movement so identified with anti-Catholicism. Historian Joseph Tregle writes that "creole support for this nativist faction foundered on the group's rabid anti-Catholic stance," and it soon collapsed locally. Joseph G. Tregle, Jr., "Creoles and Americans," in *Creole New Orleans: Race and Americanization,* ed. Arnold R. Hirsch and Joseph Logsdon (Baton Rouge: LSU Press, 1992), 166–67.

35. Randall M. Miller, "A Church in Cultural Captivity: Some Speculations on Catholic Identity in the Old South," in *Catholics in the Old South: Essays on Church and Culture,* ed. Randall M. Miller and Jon L. Wakelyn (Macon, GA: Mercer University Press, 1983), 31.

36. Minutes of June 5, 1856, Poydras Home Papers.

37. Ibid.

38. In the twentieth century, the Poydras managers undeniably adopted policies that were overtly sectarian. Their notes regarding admissions decisions in these years frequently recorded a child's rejection by the simple comment, "parents Catholic." In the 1950s, they revised

their bylaws to permit none but Protestants on the board of managers, and then stipulated that the board must have a Presbyterian majority.

6. Challenges to Poydras: The Union Army and Reconstruction

1. Minutes of April 24, 1838, September 17, 1823, and January 4, 1831, Poydras Home Papers.

2. Minutes of July 16, 1840; secretary's annual report for 1842, January 16, 1843, Poydras Home Papers.

3. Charles P. Roland, "Louisiana and Secession," *Louisiana History* 65 (May 1999): 389.

4. Christopher Duncan, "Benjamin Morgan Palmer: Southern Presbyterian Divine" (Ph.D. diss., Auburn University, 2008).

5. Benjamin M. Palmer, *Thanksgiving Sermon Delivered at the First Presbyterian Church, New Orleans* (New York: G. F. Nesbitt & Co., 1861).

6. Secretary's annual report for 1861, January 16, 1862, Poydras Home Papers.

7. Minutes of March 7, 1862, April 17, 1862, and January 16, 1864, Poydras Home Papers.

8. Kate Mason Roland and Mrs. Morris L. Croxall, eds., *The Journal of Julia LeGrand, New Orleans, 1862–63* (Richmond, VA: Everett Waddey Co., 1911), 64, 190.

9. Quoted in LeeAnn Whites and Alecia P. Long, eds., *Occupied Women: Gender, Military Occupation, and the American Civil War* (Baton Rouge: LSU Press, 2009), 29–30.

10. Minutes of October 16, 1862, Poydras Home Papers.

11. Minutes of July 18, 1861, Poydras Home Papers.

12. Secretary's annual report for 1861, January 16, 1862, Poydras Home Papers.

13. Treasurer's first quarterly report, 1862, Poydras Home Papers.

14. Treasurer's annual report for 1862, January 16, 1863, Poydras Home Papers.

15. Minutes of October 11, 1863; August Jewell to Mrs. Hodgson, n.d., Poydras Home Papers.

16. Roland and Croxall, eds., *Julia LeGrand,* 119.

17. Ibid., 47–48.

18. Entry of November 12, 1862, in managers' notebook; minutes of May 19, 1864, December 15, 1864, July 20, 1865, and August 5, 1865, Poydras Home Papers.

19. Treasurer's annual report for 1863, January 16, 1864, Poydras Home Papers.

20. Minutes of July 20, 1871, Poydras Home Papers.

21. Secretary's annual reports of 1870, 1871, and 1877; minutes of May 5, 1870, October 17, 1878, and October 22, 1878, Poydras Home Papers.

22. Minutes of July 16, 1874, Poydras Home Papers.

23. Secretary's annual report for 1869, January 17, 1870, Poydras Home Papers.

24. Minutes of February 17, 1870, Poydras Home Papers.

7. *In Sickness and in Health: The Operation of the Poydras Asylum in Its First Hundred Years*

1. J. Rhodes, "Report on the Poydras Female Orphan Asylum," *Southern Medical Reports,* vol. 1 (N.p.: B. M. Norman, 1850), 241.

2. Founding manager Ann Bryant was fatally stricken by yellow fever and died in late 1817. Minutes of August 20, 1817, and September 9, 1824, Poydras Home Papers.

3. John Duffy, ed., *The Rudolph Matas History of Medicine in Louisiana* (Baton Rouge: LSU Press, 1962), 2:12.

4. Secretary's annual reports for 1820 and 1823, January 21, 1821, and January 16, 1824; minutes of November 5, 1835, and October 3, 1839, Poydras Home Papers.

5. Reports of Visiting Committee, August 31, 1853, and October 6, 1853, Poydras Home Papers.

6. Report of Visiting Committee, October 6, 1853, Poydras Home Papers.

7. Secretary's annual report for 1878, January 16, 1879, Poydras Home Papers.

8. See Duffy, ed., *Matas History,* 2:88–92, for a detailed account of the bizarre Luzenberg affair.

9. *Proceedings of the Physico-Medical Society of New Orleans in Relation to the Trial and Expulsion of Charles A. Luzenberg* (New Orleans: Physico-Medical Society of New Orleans, 1838), first quote, 24; second quote, 25.

10. Quoted in Duffy, ed., *Matas History,* 2:91.

11. Quoted ibid., 2:90.

12. Minutes of August 23, August 27, 1917, and October 18, 1917, Poydras Home Papers. The dentist Dr. Guthrie later praised the home staff for promoting good oral hygiene among the girls, writing, "The mouths of the children of the Poydras Asylum would or should put to shame the mouths in many private practices, where children have mothers, nurses, governesses, etc. to keep them clean." Haidee Meeks Guthrie, D.D.S., to Mrs. W. S. Campbell (board president), included with secretary's annual report for 1917, January 1918, Poydras Home Papers.

13. Minutes of December 5, 1918, Poydras Home Papers. Useful information about the influenza scourge is found in Nancy K. Bristow, *American Pandemic: The Lost Worlds of the 1918 Influenza Epidemic* (New York: Oxford University Press, 2012).

14. Minutes of November 1, 1832; secretary's annual report for 1837, January 21, 1838, Poydras Home Papers.

15. Periodically there had been concerns about the quality of the children's diet, as when in 1832 the home's physician informed the managers that the health of the children was suffering because of improper food. When managers discovered that staff were giving the girls one menu and themselves a better, more plentiful one, they intervened quickly to end that practice. A few years later, when a newly hired matron reported that the children received too little bread, they authorized her to begin ordering the quantity she deemed sufficient.

16. Secretary's annual report for 1847, January 17, 1848, Poydras Home Papers.

17. Minutes of November 1821, August 7, 1823, March 4, 1829, Poydras Home Papers.

18. Letter copied into minutes of February 11, 1843, Poydras Home Papers.

19. Linda Gordon, *Pitied but Not Entitled: Single Mothers and the History of Welfare, 1890–1935* (New York: Free Press, 1994), 24.

20. Secretary's quarterly report, April–June 1869, Poydras Home Papers.

21. Secretary's quarterly report, July–October 1869; secretary's annual report for 1872, January 16, 1873; minutes of September 21, 1916, Poydras Home Papers.

22. Managers' notebook, August 11, 1858, Poydras Home Papers.

23. Copy of managers' letter to Miss Rosa Bertoulin, recorded in minutes of May 11, 1840, Poydras Home Papers.

24. Copy of letter to Mrs. Henry, in minutes of April 6, 1849, Poydras Home Papers.

25. Minutes of February 22, 1817, and November 14, 1833, Poydras Home Papers.

26. Minutes of May 3, 1832, March 1, 1860, and August 3, 1865, Poydras Home Papers.

27. Minutes of December 7, 1871, and August 3, 1876, Poydras Home Papers.

28. Minutes of January 16, 1847, and February 16, 1860, Poydras Home Papers. A set of rules formulated in 1857 upon occupation of the new building on Magazine Street required "implicit obedience" and "strict discipline," but tempered that draconian-sounding mandate by noting that punishment, while sometimes necessary, should be without "undue severity." Rules for staff undertaking to punish a girl included three: "1st Never correct a child in anger; 2nd Never break a promise; and 3rd Never overlook a fault."

29. The managers did, however, reduce the roll of widows to whom they paid monthly stipends, noting that this action was "a source of grief to us, as they are poor & needy," and promising "we shall not be slow to make amends" if times should improve. Minutes of December 20, 1877, Poydras Home Papers.

30. Anonymous to "president of Poydras," September 2, 1873, Poydras Home Papers.

31. Secretary's annual report for 1880, January 17, 1881; minutes of March 12, 1903, Poydras Home Papers.

32. Secretary's annual report for 1884, January 16, 1885, Poydras Home Papers.

8. Farewell to the Old Poydras

1. Only Georgia and South Carolina failed to adopt some form of mothers' pension before the advent of the federal program Aid to Dependent Children.

2. "New Orleans Unique Juvenile Court and Its Efficient Judge," *Case and Comment: The Lawyers' Magazine* 17 (Rochester, N.Y.: Lawyers' Cooperative Co., June 1910–May 1911).

3. The minutes featured the term "unruly" seven times in three years (1913–1916) to describe girls' behavior.

4. Minutes of October 19, 1916, and July 1, 1915, Poydras Home Papers.

5. Minutes of July 3, 1941, August 7, 1941, December 9, 1941, April 2, 1942, May 6, 1943, May 4, 1944, April 6, 1944, and September 6, 1945, Poydras Home Papers.

6. Minutes of October 1, 1936, January 17, 1957, and July 17, 1947, Poydras Home Papers.

7. Timothy A. Hacsi, *Second Home: Orphan Asylums and Poor Families in America* (Cambridge, MA: Harvard University Press, 1997), 46.

8. Minutes of August 15, 1935, and March 21, 1957, Poydras Home Papers. The drastic decision to cease regular visits to the asylum stands out all the more in that the board members took that vote in March 1957, only one month after the death of longtime manager Mrs. O. J. Paul. The secretary noted that, during Mrs. Paul's forty-seven years on the board, "she brought happiness and joy to the children of Poydras Home, whom she visited weekly. She knew them all by name, was familiar with their problems, hurts, and aspirations. Realizing her love for them, many continued to visit, call her by telephone and write to her until the close of her life." But the exemplary Mrs. Paul was ninety years old and had developed her association with Poydras girls in different and bygone times.

9. Secretary's annual report for 1938, January 16, 1939, Poydras Home Papers.

10. So thoroughly in control was John B. Ferguson that when, in 1940, he negotiated a settlement with a deadbeat tenant who owed Poydras $400 in back rent, he was incensed that the women balked at accepting it. He had agreed to take only $80 for the debt. Ferguson wrote an irate letter indicating that he felt the managers questioned his honor if they hesitated to accept his arrangements. John B. Ferguson to Mrs. O. J. Paul, January 1, 1940, Poydras Home Papers.

11. U.S. Census Bureau, "Report on Benevolent Institutions" (Washington, DC: Government Printing Office, 1910), 22.

12. Minutes of July 3, 1941, Poydras Home Papers.

13. Case notes by Mrs. Riche, matron, December 1937, Box 12, Poydras Home Papers.

14. Minutes of July 20, 1950, and August 24, 1950, Poydras Home Papers.

15. Minutes of December 6, 1956; president's annual report for 1956, January 17, 1957, Poydras Home Papers.

16. Minutes of October 20, 1955, February 15, 1951, and September 1, 1955, Poydras Home Papers.

17. The French Camp Academy, located in rural isolation near a Mississippi hamlet of fewer than two hundred people, was initially organized in 1915 by Scotch-Irish Presbyterians to serve youth from "broken" homes and troubled, dysfunctional backgrounds. Since 1950, this Christian boarding school has been governed by an interdenominational board of trustees.

18. Memo in Box 14 concerns nomenclature for the institution. Minutes of June 4, 1942, Poydras Home Papers, show that managers voted to have the word "ASYLUM" removed from the home's old iron gate.

19. Text of letter is found in minutes of November 21, 1957, Poydras Home Papers. By this time, only one Poydras girl was a full orphan. She attended Holmes Junior College in Mississippi,

with her tuition paid by the board of managers. Even after the closing of the children's home, they continued to finance her education until, at age nineteen, she left college and married.

9. And Welcome to the New!

1. Minutes of July 31, 1958; president's annual report for 1959, January 21, 1960, Poydras Home Papers. A photo of the extensive structural changes in progress appeared in the *New Orleans Times-Picayune,* March 17, 1959, 15.

2. Minutes of December 4, 1958, and January 15, 1959, Poydras Home Papers; Marion Lyons to Martha G. Robinson, May 6, 1959, in "Poydras correspondence," Collection #457, Box 1, Louisiana Research Collection, Tulane University.

3. Diane Farrell, "An Old Home Gets a New Job," *Times-Picayune Dixie Roto,* February 14, 1959, 154–55.

4. Minutes of March 17, 1960, May 5, 1960, and June 7, 1962; revised constitution of Poydras Home, c. 1960, Poydras Home Papers.

5. Minutes of January 17, 1963, Poydras Home Papers.

6. This was Joel (Mrs. Bert) Myers, a local physician's wife and Newcomb College graduate who had just earned a master's degree at Tulane and was looking for "interesting" work now that her children were no longer young. Learning that the Poydras Home needed an administrator, she applied, won the position, and subsequently stood for and passed the state licensing examination in 1979.

7. President's annual report for 1965, January 20, 1966, Poydras Home Papers. This policy was amended in 1986 to allow for the admission of Catholics and Jews.

8. Minutes of July 23, 1969, Poydras Home Papers

9. Minutes of January 24, 1966, Poydras Home Papers.

10. For information about the "Poydras boom," as well as all other developments of recent history covered in this chapter, I have relied heavily on the *New Orleans Times-Picayune,* which was for 175 years an excellent urban daily newspaper. In 2012, the paper began a new and altered life by expanding its presence as an "online platform," shrinking its able staff of reporters and photographers, and curtailing home delivery.

11. Minutes of June 16, 1966, Poydras Home Papers.

12. President's annual report for 1971, January 20, 1972, Poydras Home Papers.

13. Minutes of November 17, 1994, Poydras Home Papers.

14. Minutes of February 16, 1995, and March 8, 1995, Poydras Home Papers.

15. President's annual report for 1986, January 20, 1987; minutes of January 16, 1992, Poydras Home Papers.

16. Minutes of July 17, 1980, Poydras Home Papers.

17. Executive director's report to the board, October 17, 1996, Poydras Home Papers.

18. Minutes of November 24, 1997, Poydras Home Papers.

19. Dr. Gordon Whyte to board of managers, September 17, 1992, Poydras Home Papers.

As an example of the board's overinvolvement in minutiae, Dr. Whyte mentioned their protracted decision making over how and when to remove a storm-downed tree from the grounds of the Poydras Home. He observed that it was not complicated, should have been the administrator's responsibility, and should have been done within a few days at most. Instead, it took weeks because the managers handled it themselves.

20. Mary Langlois to "members of the Board of Administrators," September 7, 1989, and June 22, 1996, Poydras Home Papers.

21. A majority of the population heeded Mayor Nagin's urgent call and fled the city in private automobiles. The nightmarish traffic gridlock that resulted as they inched their way out of the state on clogged interstate highways led many to resolve "never again."

22. Author interview with Connie Brown, March 14, 2013, New Orleans. Fortunately, the only pets living at Poydras in 2005 were two goldfish in one resident's room, and their evacuation did not seem remotely necessary when all expected a three-day sojourn. Miraculously, when the Poydras contingent returned after two months, the finny pair were somehow still alive in the few inches of murky water that remained in their tank, seemingly emblematic of the gritty determination of the Poydras Home, its residents, staff, and managers.

23. Author interview with Sharon King, March 14, 2013, New Orleans.

24. Jed Horne, *Breach of Faith: Hurricane Katrina and the Near Death of a Great American City* (New York: Random House, 2008), 43. Various books detail the Katrina epic; I judge Horne's to be by far the best account.

25. Staffers still chuckle fondly at the affinity of some residents for alcohol. For example, when asked by a nurse's aide one Sunday afternoon, "Do you want to hear some hymns?" one hearing-impaired resident responded emphatically, "Do I want to have some gin? Yes, I want to have some gin!"

26. Author interview with Donald Dunn, March 14, 2013, New Orleans.

27. After bouncing around from place to place, Rivé settled his wife and children, ages five and three, in a house in Gonzales. Dunn and his wife obtained a place in Donaldsonville. Once Poydras reopened, he commuted down and back, a drive of seventy miles each way, for over a year while waiting for permanent housing in New Orleans.

28. Eric Lipton, "Committee Focuses on Failure to Aid New Orleans Infirm," *New York Times,* February 1, 2006. Dr. Kevin Stephens, director of the New Orleans Health Department, testified before a congressional committee in 2006 about his conversation with a local nursing home owner who told Stephens that it had cost $100,000 to evacuate his facility. He had been through earlier evacuations when the approaching hurricanes did not actually hit, after which he learned that FEMA policy prohibited any reimbursement unless the hurricane was judged to have hit the facility in question. Understandably, as Katrina blustered in the Gulf, many nursing home operators hesitated, paralyzed by a mixture of motives: an excess of caution, a reluctance to absorb the cost of moving their population needlessly, and a parallel reluctance to put the residents through the ordeal of what might be an unnecessary evacuation. "Testimony of Kevin U. Stephens, M.D.," *Challenges in a Catastrophe: Evacuating New Orleans in Advance of Hurricane Katrina* (Washington, DC: U.S. Printing Office, 2006), 31–33.

29. Anne Hull and Doug Struck, "At Nursing Home, Katrina Dealt Only the First Blow," *Washington Post,* September 23, 2005; David Rohde and Shaila Dewan, "More Deaths Confirmed in Homes for the Aged," *New York Times,* September 15, 2005; Laura Parker, "What Really Happened at St. Rita's?" *USA Today,* November 28, 2005.

30. Minutes of November 17, 2005, Poydras Home Papers.

31. President's annual report for 2006, January 20, 2007; executive director's annual report for 2006, January 2007, Poydras Home Papers.

Afterword

1. I am indebted to Arlene Kaplan Daniels for the concept of the "invisible career," a term she uses to describe the unpaid but valuable work of women in voluntary associations. See Daniels, *Invisible Careers: Women Civic Leaders from the Volunteer World* (Chicago: University of Chicago Press, 1988.

2. Minutes of November 28, 1817, and secretary's annual report for 1821 [undated, early 1822], Poydras Home Papers.

3. The quotes come from secretary's annual report for 1843, February 18, 1844; and minutes of April 20, 1849, February 23, 1878, February 6, 1879, and May 5, 1881, respectively. The remark about Marmee is found in Anne Firor Scott's landmark study, *Natural Allies: Women's Associations in American History* (Urbana: University of Illinois Press, 1993), 16.

A NOTE ON SOURCES

he editors at Louisiana State University Press supported me in my decision to provide citations for direct quotations only. In this section I recognize, gratefully, the many indispensable authors who contributed information essential to the preparation of this book.

There is a small but growing literature on the history of "orphanages," those institutions that cared not only for parentless youth but also for needy and neglected children in our country's past. Of special usefulness to me was Timothy A. Hacsi's *Second Home: Orphan Asylums and Poor Families in America* (Cambridge, MA: Harvard University Press, 1997). In clear prose, Hacsi acquainted me with general trends of the nineteenth-century asylum and changed forever my understanding of such institutions. Thanks to Hacsi, I learned of the vital role these places played for millions. Though not offering the equivalent of parental love (and what large institution could do that?), they provided safety and stability and were in general a valuable resource for the poor of our country.

From Kenneth Cmiel, *A Home of Another Kind: One Chicago Orphanage and the Tangle of Child Welfare* (Chicago: University of Chicago Press, 1995), I formed my understanding of change over time in children's homes and in ideas about child welfare, making the valuable discovery that developments he tracked so carefully in Chicago had counterparts in the Poydras Asylum. Other works on orphanages that I consulted profitably include Judith A. Dulberger, *"Mother donit fore the best": Correspondence of a Nineteenth-Century Orphan Asylum* (Syracuse: Syracuse University Press, 1996), and Susan Whitelaw Downs and Michael W. Sherraden, "The Orphan Asylum in the Nineteenth Century," *Social Service Review* 57 (June 1983): 272–90. From Matthew A. Crenson, *Building the Invisible Orphanage: A Prehistory of the American Wel-*

fare System (Cambridge, MA: Harvard University Press, 2009), I learned about the pivotal "child-rescue movement" of the early twentieth century. Linda Gordon, *Pitied but Not Entitled: Single Mothers and the History of Welfare, 1890–1935* (New York: Free Press, 1994), is a sweeping analysis that had significant bearing on my understanding of both the role of orphanages and the changing attitudes of policymakers toward single mothers, whether widowed, deserted, divorced, or never married.

Several essays in *Children Bound to Labor: The Pauper Apprentice System in Early America* (Ithaca: Cornell University Press, 2009), edited by Ruth Wallis Herndon and John E. Murray, were valuable for this project. I will mention Paul LaChance's essay on indentured children's literacy in New Orleans, Timothy J. Lockley's work on children bound out in Savannah, and Monique Bourque's article on the practice of apprenticing children in Chester County, Pennsylvania, the very spot from which Poydras Asylum founder Phoebe Hunter hailed. John E. Murray is also the author of the excellent close study *The Charleston Orphan House: Children's Lives in the First Public Orphanage in America* (Chicago: University of Chicago Press, 2013). Homer Folks, *The Care of Destitute, Neglected, and Delinquent Children* (New York: Macmillan, 1902), is a classic by the prominent sociologist who worked with children's aid societies one hundred years ago.

Anne Firor Scott's graceful synthesis, *Natural Allies: Women's Associations in American History* (Urbana: University of Illinois Press, 1991), is bursting with insights about the rich history of women's benevolent work. Lori D. Ginzberg, *Women and the Work of Benevolence: Morality, Politics, and Class in the Nineteenth-Century United States* (New Haven: Yale University Press, 1990), was also valuable for a penetrating look at women's charitable work outside the South. Patricia Ferguson Clement, "Children and Charity: Orphanages in New Orleans, 1817–1914," *Louisiana History* 27 (Autumn 1986): 337–51; Gail S. Murray, "Charity within the Bounds of Race and Class: Female Benevolence in the Old South," *South Carolina Historical Magazine* 96 (January 1995): 54–70; and Elna C. Green's essay "National Trends, Regional Differences, Local Circumstances: Social Welfare in New Orleans, 1870s–1920s," in her edited volume *Before the New Deal: Social Welfare in the South, 1830–1930* (Athens: University of Georgia Press, 1999), are all useful for information on white women's benevolence in New Orleans. Another scholar's work in dissertation form that proved helpful was Jonathan David Sarnoff, "White Women and Respectability in Antebellum New Orleans, 1830–1861," Ph.D. diss., University of Southern Mississippi, 2003.

In secondary research for the expedition of Dunbar and Hunter, I relied primarily on *The Forgotten Expedition, 1804–1805: The Louisiana Purchase Journals of Dunbar and Hunter*, ed. Trey Berry, Pam Beasley, and Jeanne Clements (Baton Rouge: LSU Press, 2006). Biographical information on George Hunter comes from this and from Patrick G. Williams, S. Charles Bolton, and Jeannie M. Whayne, eds., *A Whole Country in Commotion: The Louisiana Purchase and the American Southwest* (Fayetteville: University of Arkansas Press, 2005). My understanding of New Orleans in its first decades comes largely from Lawrence N. Powell's fascinating and authoritative account, *The Accidental City: Improvising New Orleans* (Cambridge, MA: Harvard University Press, 2012), supplemented by Peter J. Kastor, *The Nation's Crucible: The Louisiana Purchase and the Creation of America* (New Haven: Yale University Press, 2004). The prolific Richard Campanella's works aided me as I attempted to understand the expansion of New Orleans beyond its origins in the French Quarter, particularly *Bienville's Dilemma: A Historical Geography of New Orleans* (Lafayette: Center for Louisiana Studies, University of Louisiana at Lafayette, 2008) and *Time and Place in New Orleans: Past Geographies in the Present Day* (Gretna: Pelican Publishing, 2002). B. B. Edwards, *Memoir of the Rev. Elias Cornelius* (Boston: Perkins and Marvin, 1833), was a useful primary source for this early period.

For an understanding of Phoebe Bryant Hunter and the specific cultural and religious forces that shaped her, I consulted several sources: Margaret Hope Bacon, *Mothers of Feminism: The Story of Quaker Women in America* (San Francisco: Harper & Row, 1986); Rosemary Abend, "Constant Samaritans: Quaker Philanthropy in Philadelphia, 1680–1799," Ph.D. diss., University of California–Los Angeles, 1988; Margaret Morris Haviland, "Beyond Women's Sphere: Young Quaker Women and the Veil of Charity in Philadelphia, 1790–1810," *William & Mary Quarterly* 51 (July 1994): 419–46; and Bruce Dorsey, "Friends Becoming Enemies: Philadelphia Benevolence and the Neglected Era of American Quaker History," *Journal of the Early Republic* 18 (Autumn 1998): 395–428.

I owe a very special debt to Mark Duvall, who has researched and published material on the earliest years of the Poydras Asylum and on founder Phoebe Hunter. I read both his master's thesis and an article still in manuscript form with pleasure: Mark Duvall, "The New Orleans Female Orphan Society: Labor, Education, and Americanization, 1817–1833," M.A. thesis, University of New Orleans, 2009, and Duvall, "Phoebe Hunter, 1760–1844: Neither Northern nor Southern," in *Louisiana Women*, vol. 2, ed. Shannon Frystak (Athens: University of Georgia Press, 2015). Duvall dug deep into manuscript sources for the Monthly Meeting of Women's Friends, Southern District of Philadelphia, 1787, housed in Haverford College Special Collections; his findings there revealed some key aspects of Hunter's early life.

Sources that were essential for chapter 3 include Emily Clark, *Masterless Mistresses: The New Orleans Ursulines and the Development of a New World Society, 1727–1834* (Chapel Hill: University of North Carolina Press, 2007); Brian J. Costello, *The Life, Family and Legacy of Julien Poydras* (N.p.: John and Noelie Laurent Ewing, 2001); Gwendolyn Midlo Hall, *Africans in Colonial Louisiana: The Development of Afro-Creole Culture in the Eighteenth Century* (Baton Rouge: LSU Press, 1992); Christina Vella, *Intimate Enemies: The Two Worlds of the Baroness de Pontalba* (Baton Rouge: LSU Press, 1997); and Paul LaChance, "The 1809 Immigration of Saint-Domingue Refugees to New Orleans: Reception, Integration and Impact," *Louisiana History* 29 (Spring 1988): 109–41.

Information on the complex legacies of Alexander Milne and Stephen Henderson comes from Francis P. Burns, "The Fortune That Disappeared," *Times-Picayune Dixie Roto,* September 24, 1950; Judith K. Schafer, *Slavery, the Civil Law, and the Supreme Court of Louisiana* (Baton Rouge: LSU Press, 1994); and Roulhac Toledano et al. *New Orleans Architecture,* vol. 6: *Faubourg Tremé and the Bayou Road* (Gretna: Pelican Publishing, 2003). Good sources for understanding female education in Louisiana in the nineteenth century were Dolores E. Labbe, "Women in Early Nineteenth-Century Louisiana," Ph.D. diss., University of Delaware, 1975; and Thomas G. Conway, "John A. Kennicott: A Teacher in New Orleans," *Louisiana History* 26 (Autumn 1985): 399–415; as well as Emily Clark's account of the work of the Ursulines, *Masterless Mistresses*. A description of the monitorial approach, which Poydras managers ultimately declined to employ, is delivered in William R. Johnson, "'Chanting Cloisters': Simultaneous Recitation in Baltimore's Nineteenth-Century Primary Schools," *History of Education Quarterly 34* (Spring 1994): 1–23.

Unraveling the fascinating tale of religious strife at the asylum led me to read a variety of sources. Rebecca Reed, *Six Months in a Convent, or the Nar-*

rative of Rebecca Theresa Reed Who Was Under the Influence of Roman Catholics about two years and an inmate of the Ursuline convent on Mount Benedict in Charlestown, Mass. Nearly Six Months in the Years 1831–32 (Boston: Russell, Odiorne and Metcalf, 1835), and Maria Monk, *Awful Disclosures of Maria Monk, as exhibited in a narrative of her sufferings during a residence of five years as a novice, and two years as a black nun in the Hotel Dieu nunnery at Montreal* ... (New York: Howe & Bates, 1836), are the two inflammatory works that intensified the anti-Catholic backlash of the 1830s. Two articles by Susan M. Griffin, "Awful Disclosures: Women's Evidence in the Escaped Nun's Tale," *PMLA* 111 (January 1996): 93–107; and "'The Dark Stranger': Sensationalism and Anti-Catholicism in Sarah Josepha Hale's *Traits of American Life*," *Legacy* 14 (1997): 13–24, illuminated themes foregrounded by those works and explained the reaction of many Americans. Jenny Franchot, *Roads to Rome: The Antebellum Protestant Encounter with Catholicism* (Berkeley: University of California Press, 1994), is an excellent source for insights into the religious tensions that gripped antebellum America, as is an older but still solid work by Ray A. Billington, *The Protestant Crusade, 1800–1860: A Study of the Origins of American Nativism* (New York: Rinehart, 1938). For an understanding of the outlook of Catholics in Protestant America in the nineteenth century, John O'Grady, *Catholic Charities in the United States: History and Problems* (Washington DC: National Conference of Catholic Charities, 1931), was informative. Information about key differences between the views and practices of Latin, or Creole, Catholics and Irish Catholics is found in essays in *Catholics in the Old South: Essays on Church and Culture,* edited by Randall M. Miller and Jon L. Wakelyn (Macon, GA: Mercer University Press, 1983), especially the pieces by Miller, "A Church in Cultural Captivity: Some Speculations on Catholic Identity in the Old South," 11–52, and Dennis Clark, "The South's Irish Catholics: A Case of Cultural Confinement," 195–209. I gained understanding of the practices of the Sisters of Charity from Mary Ewens, O.P., "The Role of the Nun in Nineteenth-Century America," Ph.D. diss., University of Minnesota, 1971. Other useful sources for gaining a grasp of the religious landscape in New Orleans were Julia McGowan, "The Presbyterian Churches in New Orleans during Reconstruction," M.A. thesis, Tulane University, 1930; Louis Voss, *The Beginnings of Presbyterianism in the Southwest* (New Orleans: Presbyterian Board of Publications of the Synod of Louisiana, 1923); Theodore Clapp,

Autobiographical Sketches and Recollections: During a Thirty-Five Years' Resi-dence in New Orleans (Boston: Phillips, Sampson & Co., 1857); and Timothy Reilly, "Parson Clapp of New Orleans: Antebellum Social Critic, Religious Rad-ical and Member of the Establishment," *Louisiana History* 16 (Spring 1975): 167–91. I also consulted manuscript sources, including correspondence be-tween various nuns and their superiors and between Father Adam Kindelon and his bishop, housed at the Office of Archives and Records, Archdiocese of New Orleans, where Dorenda Dupont proved accommodating and knowl-edgeable. Understanding the complex ethnic realities of antebellum New Orleans necessitated grasping the struggle between Creoles and Americans, beautifully illuminated in Joseph G. Tregle, Jr.'s important essay "Creoles and New Orleans," in *Creole New Orleans: Race and Americanization,* edited by Ar-nold R. Hirsch and Joseph Logsdon (Baton Rouge: LSU Press, 1992), 131–85.

Sectionalism, the Civil War, and Reconstruction have long commanded the attention of historians. For the Louisiana experience, see John M. Sacher, "The Sudden Collapse of the Louisiana Whig Party," *Journal of Southern His-tory* 65 (May 1999): 221–48, and Charles P. Roland, "Louisiana and Secession," *Louisiana History* 19 (Autumn 1978): 389–99. Christopher Duncan, "Benja-min Morgan Palmer: Southern Presbyterian Divine," Ph.D. diss., Auburn Uni-versity, 2008, and Benjamin M. Palmer, *Thanksgiving Sermon Delivered at the First Presbyterian Church, New Orleans* (New York: G. F. Nesbitt & Co., 1861), illuminated the fire-breathing pastor in whose congregation many Poydras managers sat. The musings of the unhappy southerner Julia LeGrand, who spent part of the war in New Orleans, were published in *The Journal of Julia LeGrand, New Orleans, 1862–63,* ed. Kate Mason Rowland and Mrs. Morris L. Croxall (Richmond, VA: Everett Waddey Co., 1911). For a full analysis of General Butler's infamous order, which emphasizes his failure to subjugate Confederate women in New Orleans, see Alecia P. Long, "(Mis)Remember-ing General Order No. 28: Benjamin Butler, the Woman Order, and Historical Memory," in *Occupied Women: Gender, Military Occupation, and the American Civil War,* ed. LeeAnn Whites and Alecia P. Long (Baton Rouge: LSU Press, 2009). For knowledge of New Orleans in Reconstruction, I relied on Justin A. Nystrom, *New Orleans after the Civil War: Race, Politics, and a New Birth of Freedom* (Baltimore: Johns Hopkins University Press, 2010); James G. Hol-landsworth, *An Absolute Massacre: The New Orleans Race Riot of July 30, 1866*

(Baton Rouge: LSU Press, 2001); and James K. Hogue, *Uncivil War: Five New Orleans Street Battles and the Rise and Fall of Radical Reconstruction* (Baton Rouge: LSU Press, 2006).

The chief sources for my conclusions about matters of health at Poydras were works by two prominent medical historians: Charles E. Rosenberg, *The Cholera Years: The United States in 1832, 1849, and 1866* (1962; Chicago: University of Chicago Press, 1987); John Duffy, ed., *The Rudolph Matas History of Medicine in Louisiana*, vol. 2 (Baton Rouge: LSU Press, 1962); and John Duffy, *From Humors to Medical Science: A History of American Medicine* (Urbana: University of Illinois Press, 1994). Other useful works include Jo Ann Carrigan, *The Saffron Scourge: A History of Yellow Fever in Louisiana, 1796–1905* (Lafayette: Center for Louisiana Studies, University of Southwestern Louisiana, 1994), John Salvaggio, *New Orleans' Charity Hospital: A Story of Physicians, Politics, and Poverty* (Baton Rouge: LSU Press, 1992), and Nancy K. Bristow, *American Pandemic: The Lost Worlds of the 1918 Influenza Epidemic* (Oxford: Oxford University Press, 2012). Something close to comic relief was found in *Proceedings of the Physico-Medical Society of New Orleans in Relation to the Trial and Expulsion of Charles A. Luzenberg* (New Orleans: Physico-Medical Society of New Orleans, 1838), detailing the bizarre episode of Dr. Luzenberg's disgrace.

Some admirable research, much of it conducted in New Orleans, aided me in understanding the rise of public welfare and the changing nature of the orphanage in the twentieth century. Elizabeth Wisner, longtime dean of Tulane's School of Social Work, wrote "The Louisiana Law of Family Relations," *Social Service Review* 3 (December 1929): 584–96, and *Public Welfare Administration in Louisiana* (Chicago: University of Chicago Press, 1930). Valuable theses and dissertations concerning public welfare in Louisiana include Julianna Liles Boudreaux, "A History of Philanthropy in New Orleans, 1835–1862," Ph.D. diss., Tulane University, 1961; Robert Earl Moran, "The History of Child Welfare in Louisiana, 1850–1960," Ph.D. diss., Ohio State University, 1968; Gladys Soulé, "The History of the Family Services Society of New Orleans," M.S. thesis, Tulane University, 1947; and Jamie Jackson Payne, "A History of the New Orleans Hospital and Dispensary for Women and Children," M.S.W. thesis, Tulane University, 1947. Also useful was Evelyn Campbell Beven, *City Subsidies in Private Charitable Agencies in New Orleans: The History and Present Status, 1824–1933* (New Orleans: School of Social Work, Tulane University, 1934).

For understanding the past fifty years in New Orleans, I relied most heavily on the *New Orleans Times-Picayune,* which boasts a long, proud history as one of the nation's premier urban dailies. Year after year, its ample staff of talented reporters and photographers detailed local events with accuracy and panache, their legacy of crackling prose and memorable images educating me on every aspect of this city and allowing me to enjoy the process all the way. Oral history also played a significant part as I strove to report recent history at the Poydras Home. Phoebe Hunter's descendant Hunter Babin talked with me about his illustrious ancestor. Past and present members of the Poydras staff sat for interviews, offering enlightening vignettes and details and, in particular, bringing the Katrina experience to life. Joel G. Myers, Jay Rivé, Sharon King, Donald Dunn, and Connie Brown were generous with their time and articulate in their recollections. So too were Poydras board members Mary Langlois, Pat Rosamond, Nelda Sibley, and Karen G. Smith, who made vivid for me the deep feelings they share for that venerable institution on Magazine Street.

INDEX

Note: Italics indicate pages with illustrations.